Recipes Of Ital

4 books in 1

A Collection Of 4 Different Cookbooks With All The Best Recipes Of The Italian Tradition

Charlie Sims - Italian Academy Of Cuisine

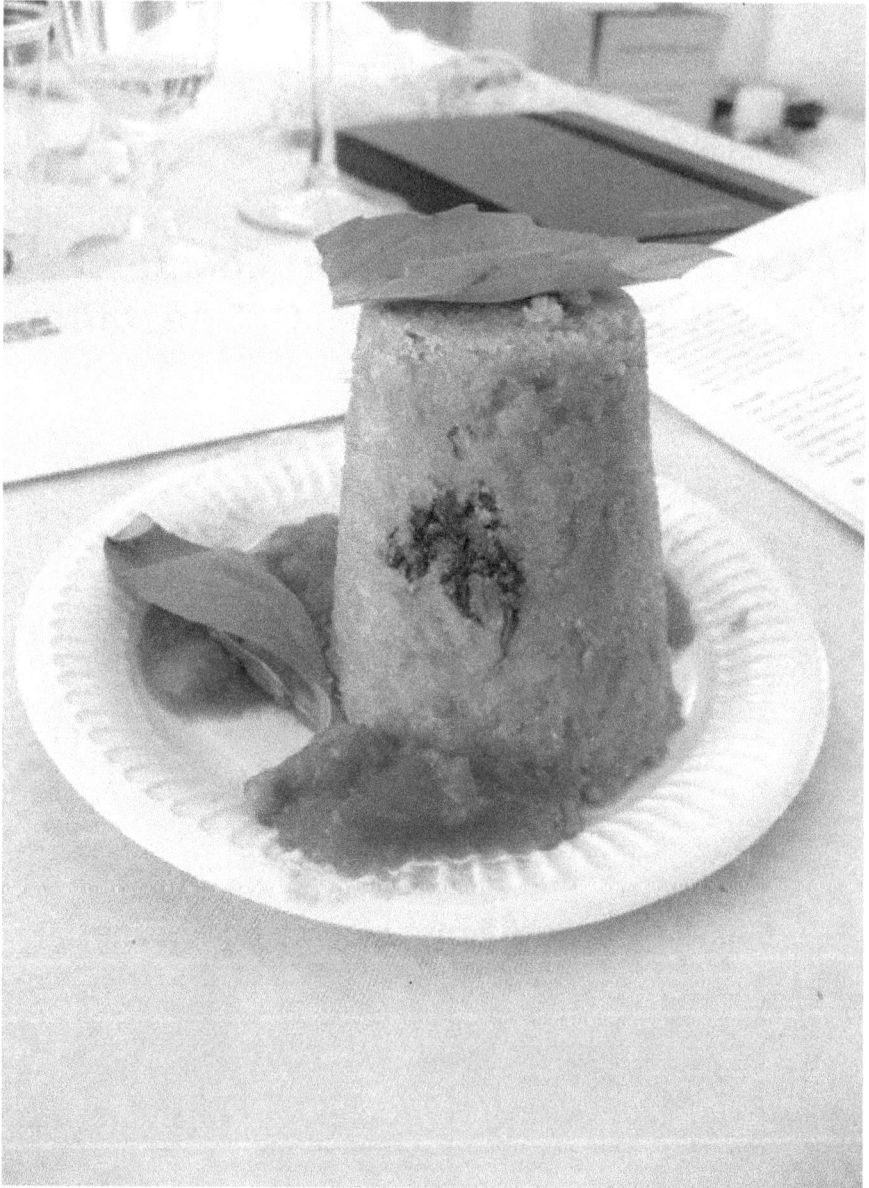

Stuffed Tomatoes

Ingredients:

- 4 tomatoes
- 2 goat cheeses
- Basil
- Salt
- white pepper

Description:

Cut the tomatoes in half horizontally, empty all halves of the pulp that you will keep aside, salt the cups obtained and let them rest a little upside down with the hollow underneath.

Mince the pulp removed from the tomatoes, put it in a bowl with a little salt and a pinch of freshly ground pepper and add the goat cheese.

Work everything with a fork to obtain a homogeneous mixture, wash the basil, finely chop the leaves and incorporate them into the cheese mixture.

Stuff the half-tomatoes with the prepared stuffing and arrange them on a serving plate garnished with salad leaves.

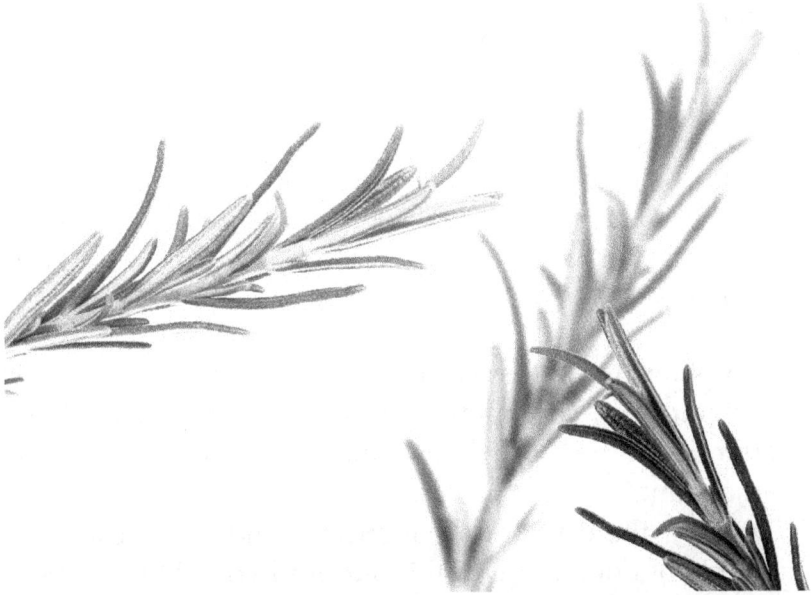

Tigelle

Ingredients:

- 250g flour0
- 500g flour 00
- 300g milk
- 200g water
- 60g lard
- oil
- Dry yeast
- salt

Description:

in a planetary mixer, combine the 2 flours and the milk with the dry yeast, operate the machine and add the lard, after 1 minute, add the oil and water, when it is well amalgamated add the salt.

Transfer the dough onto a surface and let it rest for a couple of hours. now roll it out until you obtain a sheet of half a cm, with a circular shape, make as many tigelle as

possible, let it rest for 30 minutes and cook it in a pan for 5 minutes on each side. If they are still white, continue until they are nicely colored.

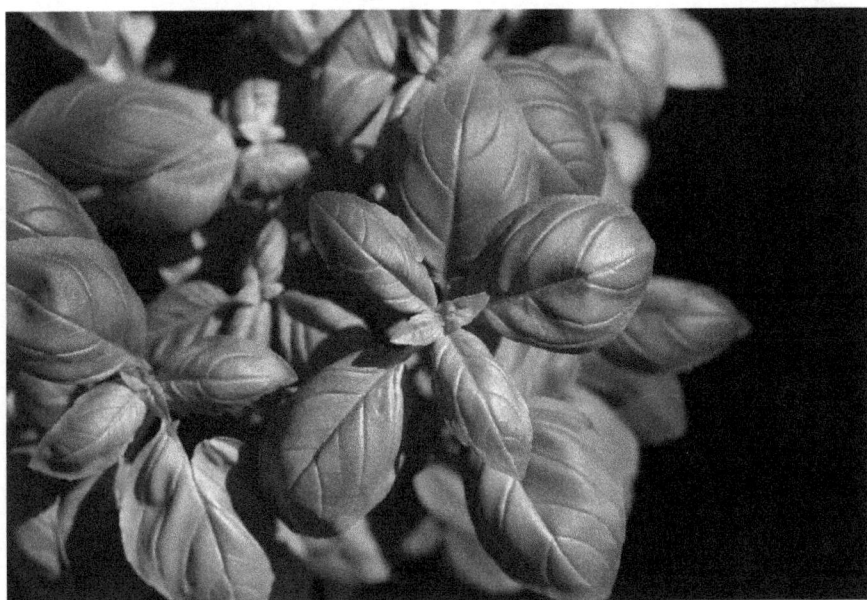

Caramelized Onions

Ingredients:

- 1kg onions
- 70g sugar
- 80g brown sugar
- 250g water

Description:

tagliare tutte le cipolle e onetele inuna casservuola e aggiungere subito i due zuccheri, successivamente anche l'acqua, lasciate a fuoco moderato per 1 ora circa, di tanto in tanto mescolate. Da servire su crostini o come contorno per carni.

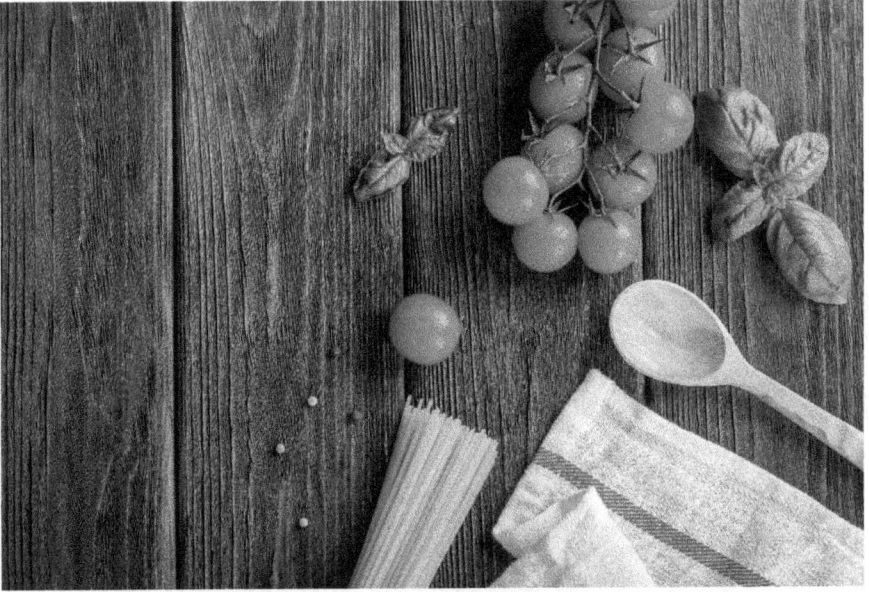

baked squid

Ingredients:

- 600g squid
- 200g breadcrumbs
- 20g paprika
- Oil and salt

Description:

Take the squid wash and clean them, creating rings with the body of the squid. Separately, in a bowl, put breadcrumbs and paprika with salt, place the mixture in a baking dish and pour the rings with the tentacles, flour them well and then, after lining a baking dish with parchment paper, place the fish on top with a turn of olive oil. Bake for 25 minutes at 180°.

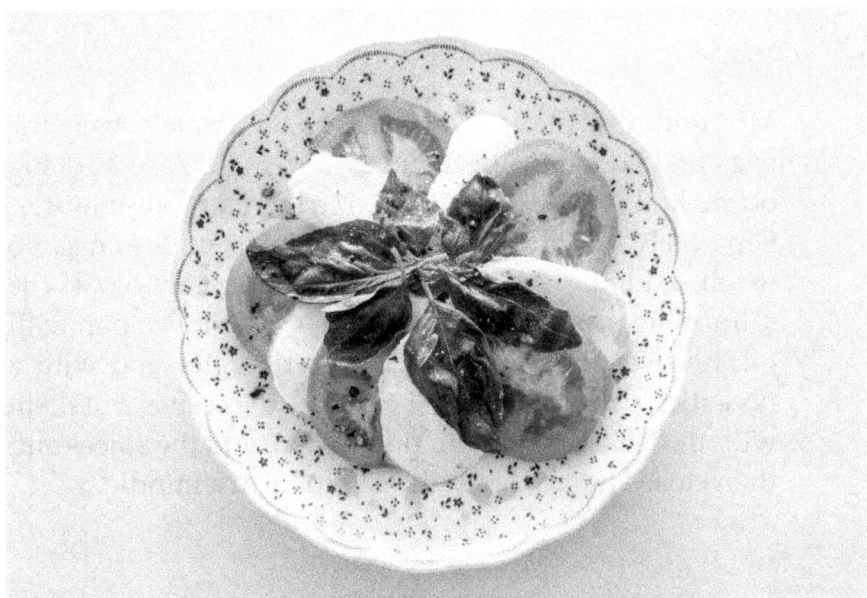

Surprise casket

Ingredients:

2 eggs, 300g milk, 150g garina00, 40g butter, salt, 500g leeks, 100g robiola, 100g salmon, grated grana cheese, nutmeg, salt, pepper, thyme, garlic

Description:

Mix milk and flour with a whisk, separately beat the eggs and add them to the flour and milk. Also add 40g of melted butter. Leave in refrigerator 30 minutes. Separately, cut the leeks into very thin rounds and sauté in oil, add the milk and thyme. Separately, cook the salmon steak already cut into cubes, pass it in a pan with oil. Recover the mixture in the refrigerator and with a non-stick pan, you're going to create the crepes. Fill them with the leek mixture and the salmon, add the spices and then close and tie the creps as if to form a bundle.

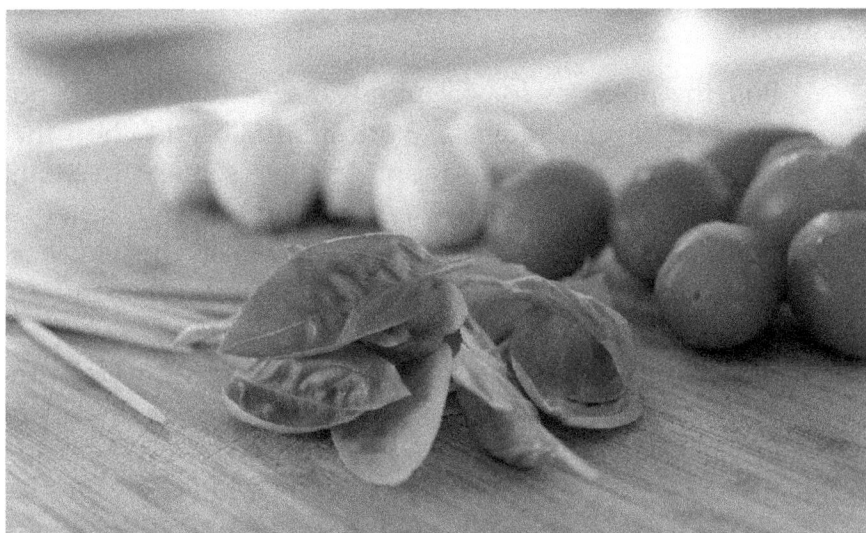

Sausage and Potato Pie

Ingredients:

600g potatoes, 1 egg, 100g granan, 200g cornstarch, 360g sausage, 550g buffalo mozzarella, 1 shallot, rosemary salt and pepper.

Description:

Boil the potatoes for 45 minutes, slice the buffalo and drain it in a colander, leave the buffalo and chop the shallot and gut the sausage, chop the rosemary. In a pan with oil, add shallot, rosemary and sausage, after 2 minutes add white wine, turn off as soon as the wine has evaporated. Mash the boiled potatoes with a potato masher, add

half of the grana cheese, pepper, egg and knead with your hands. Line a baking pan with a high edge with baking paper, with half of the potatoes, create the base, just

above add the drained buffalo and finally the sausage, cover with the rest of the potatoes, salt pepper and parmesan cheese. Bake for 20 minutes at 250°, cut and serve.

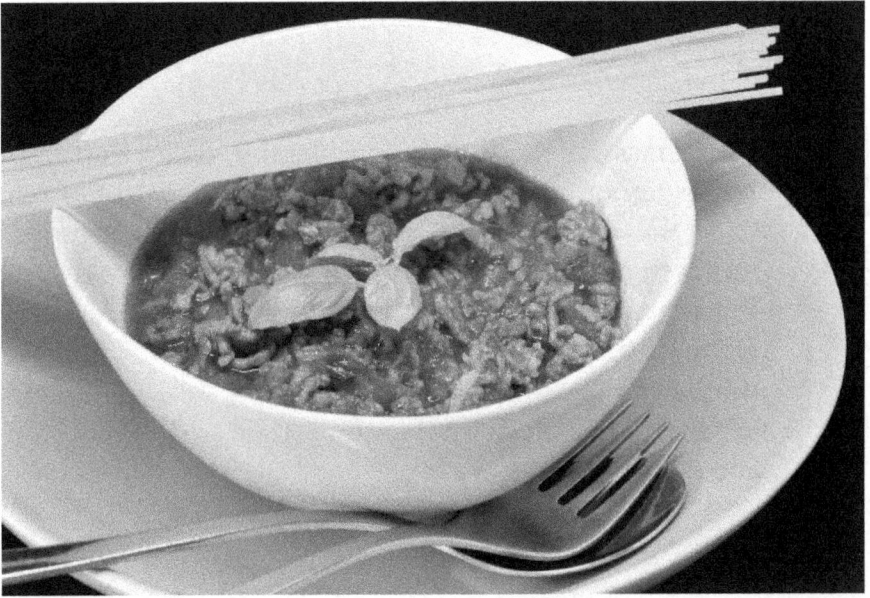

Shrimp Cocktail

Ingredients:

16 shrimps, 60g iceberg lettuce, 4 lemon slices, 1 yolk, 120g seed oil, 15g lemon juice, 45g ketchup, 1 tablespoon worcestershire sauce, tabasco brandy, salt pepper

Description:

in the glass for the immersion blender, insert yolk salt pepper lemon juice, blend and flush add the seed oil. When the mayonnaise is ready, add the ketchup and worchester sauce, tabsco and bandy and leave to rest in the fridge. Clean the shrimp, remove the carapace, head and legs. Cut the lettuce into strips and place a small amount in the designated glass, insert 4 shrimp making sure they come out with their tails, then add the cocktail sauce.

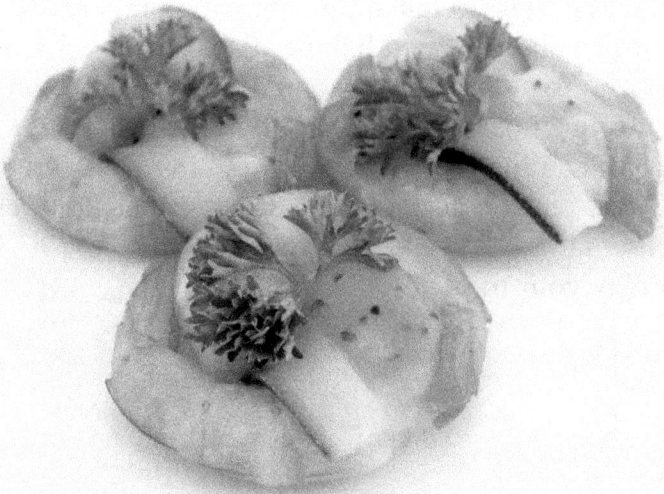

Polenta Fries

Ingredients:

250g polenta flour, 1liter water, olive oil, rosemary salt and seed oil.

Description:

Use the flour to make polenta, when it is ready, pour it into an already oiled baking dish. Let it cool around for 3-4 hours. After this time, place the polenta on a clean cutting board and begin to slice it. Creating parallelepipeds, which we are going to fry in seed oil. Once ready season with salt pepper and chopped rosemary.

Enjoy your meal

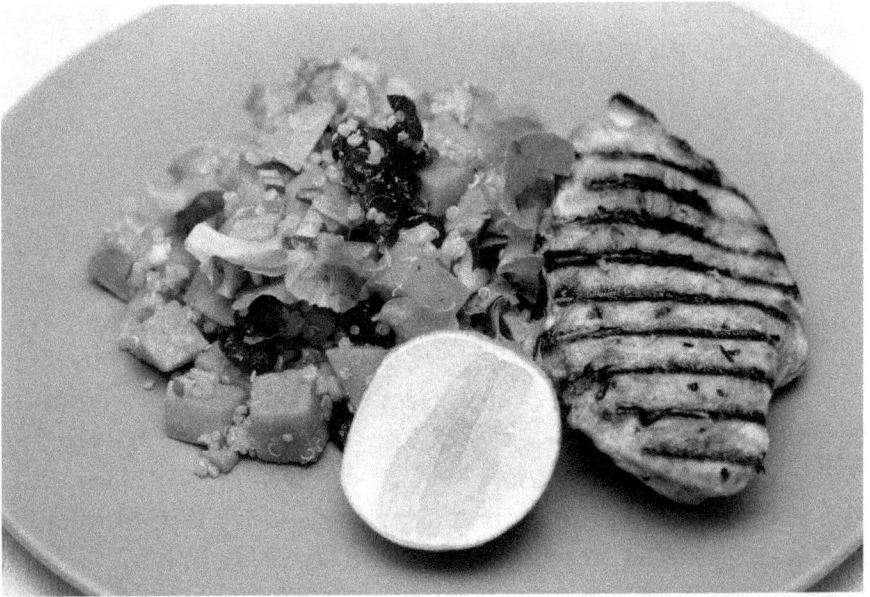

Pumpkin Poleptte

Ingredients:

- 500g pumpkin
- 100g breadcrumbs
- 100g parmesan cheese
- 50g scamorza cheese
- 1 egg
- Sage oil salt pepper

Description:

Peel the pumpkin and slice it thinly, put it in a baking pan and bake 30 minutes at 200°. Chop sage garlic and scamorza cheese. Remove the pumpkin from the oven and transfer it to a bowl, add the bread crumbs, the Parmesan cheese, the egg and the sage; create a smooth dough, take a piece of dough, create a small ball in the center of which there will be a few pieces of scamorza cheese, dip it in the breadcrumbs and fry it until it looks golden, dry your meatballs and serve them hot.

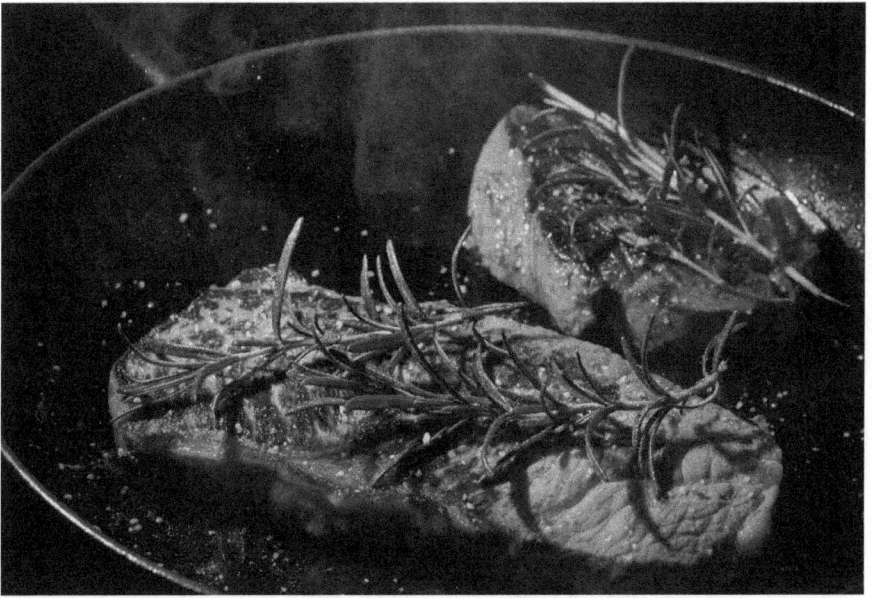

Caponata

Ingredients:

1kg eggplants, 400g celery, 250g onions, 200g tomatoes, 200g olives, 50g capers, 50g pine nuts, 60g sugar, 60g white vinegar, 40g tomato paste, basil oil salt, oil for frying

Description:

cut all the vegetables, celery onions olives eggplant tomatoes, meanwhile in a pan toast the ponoli, being careful not to burn them. Fry the eggplant in pieces, dry it and keep it aside. In a saucepan, place the oil, onion, celery, capers, olives, pine nuts, toasted tomatoes, and let everything cook for 20 minutes over low heat. In a small bowl, combine the vinegar with the tomato paste and sugar, stir and add to the saucepan, at which point add the eggplant and basil leaves. Caponata is good both hot and cold the next day.

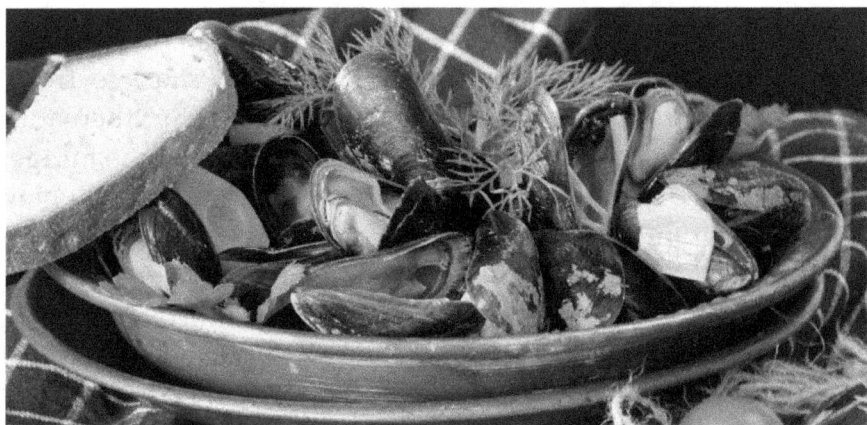

Cabbage Rolls

Ingredients:

250g rice, 6 savoy cabbage leaves, 350g sausage, 40g celery, 40g carrots, 40g onions, 50g oil, 30g butter, 1litre stock, 80g Parmesan cheese, 60g white wine, salt, pepper, thyme.

Description:

Chop onions and carrots flat. Remove sausage from casing. In a saucepan combine oil and butter, then add the chopped vegetables, after 3 minutes add the sausage paste, deglaze with white wine, add the thyme, when everything is browned, add a few ladles of hot vegetable broth, add the rice and cook it as a risotto. Separately, blanch the veza leaves to make them a little softer; each leaf will hold our rice with sausage. When all the rolls are ready, place them in an oven dish and cook for 15 minutes at 200°.

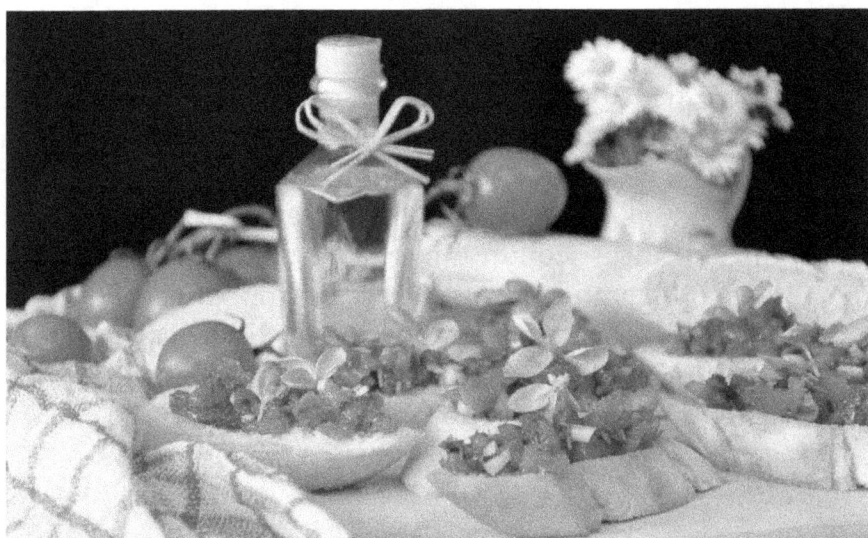

Chickpea Poleptte

Ingredients:

250g chickpeas, 60g shallot, mustard seeds, thyme, rosemary, 1 egg, oil, 130g scamorza cheese, salt and pepper. Milk breadcrumbs oil for frying.

Description:

Leave the dried chickpeas to soak for 12 hours. Then pour them into a pot with plenty of cold water. Cook for 2 hours, pour them drained into a bowl seasoned with salt and oil, mince a shallot and scamorza cheese blend the chickpeas iconun mixer with thyme, shallot, veal, egg and scamorza cheese. Once the mixture is obtained, we will have to make many meatballs, which we will pass first in the beaten egg and then in the breadcrumbs, fry and then dry with absorbent paper.

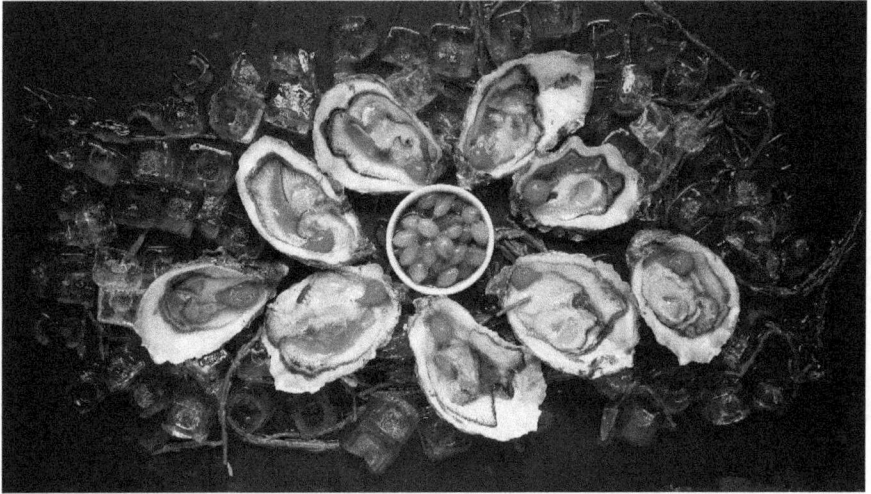

Artichokes Alla Giudia

Ingredients:

- 4 violets
- seed oil
- salt

Description:

Carefully clean the mammole, keeping the stem of 5-6 cm maximum, remove leaves until you get to the lightest ones, beat the artichoke on the cutting board upside down. Heat a saucepan with seed oil, insert an artichoke at a time, upside down, with your hands or pliers, crush the artichoke down, so as to make it similar to an open flower, after 5-6 minutes it should be cooked, turn it on its side and cook the stem. Drain it and proceed with the others.

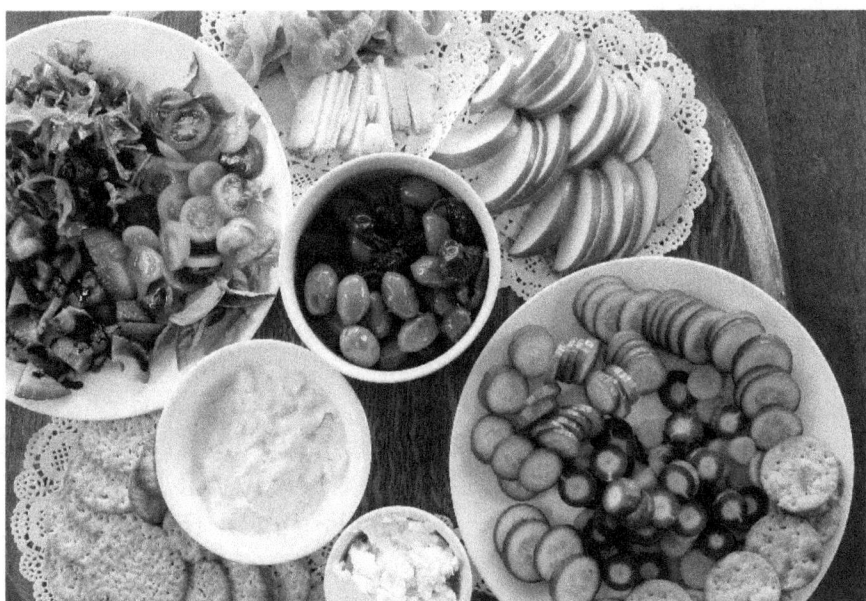

Eggplant Poleptte

Ingredients:

- 800g eggplants
- 120g breadcrumbs
- 120g parmesan cheese
- 2 eggs
- parsley
- Oil for frying
- Garlic pepper salt

Description:

Cut the eggplants in half lengthwise, place in a 200° static oven for 50 minutes. Once cool, peel off the skin. With a strainer, squeeze the pulp removing all the remaining liquid; put the pulp in a bowl and add the eggs and crushed garlic. Combine the two compounds and knead with your hands, when it will be smooth, begin to form the meatballs; pass them in the breadcrumbs and then in hot oil (for a good frying, the ideal temperature is 170 °).

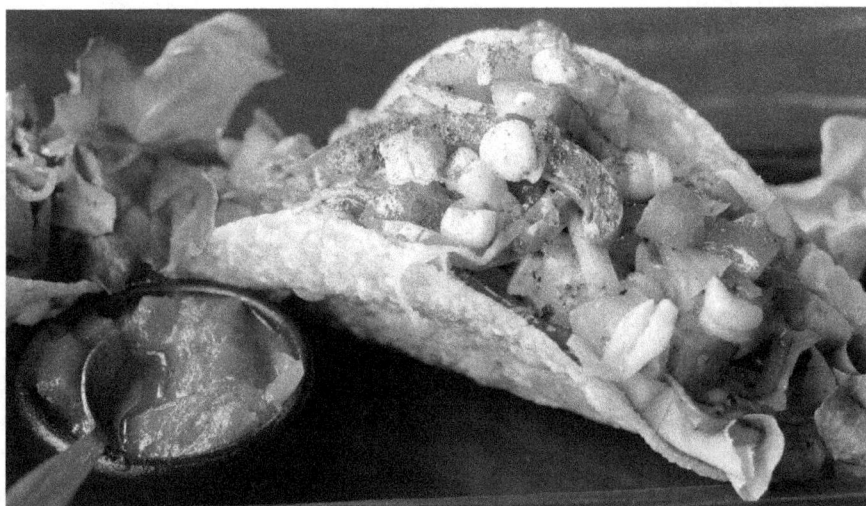

Asparagus In Crust

Ingredients:

- 800g asparagus
- 250g puff pastry
- 8 slices of raw ham
- 30g Parmesan cheese
- 1 egg

Description:

clean and boil the asparagus for 10 minutes, roll out a sheet of puff pastry and cut it into 3cm strips. Wrap the asparagus with the prosciutto and then with one of the cut strips, creating a spiral, brush each asparagus with egg yolk 15 minutes at 200° in the oven and they will be ready to serve.

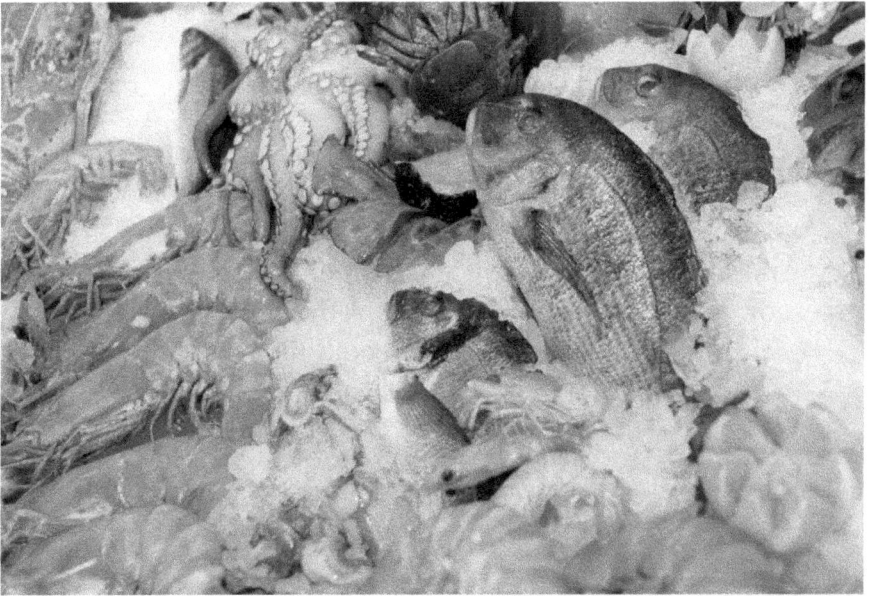

Frittata Of Zucchini

Ingredients:

eggs, nutmeg, grana cheese, zucchini, oil, garlic, salt, pepper.

Description:

Cut the zucchinis into rounds, add salt and pepper, add the oil in a frying pan with a clove of garlic, remove the garlic and add the cut zucchinis. Separately, prepare the eggs, beat them and slowly add the grttato bread, grana cheese, salt and nutmeg. When everything is well amalgamated, add the zucchini to the pan, using a plate or lid, grate the omelette, remember to eat it hot, although it will also be good cold the next day!

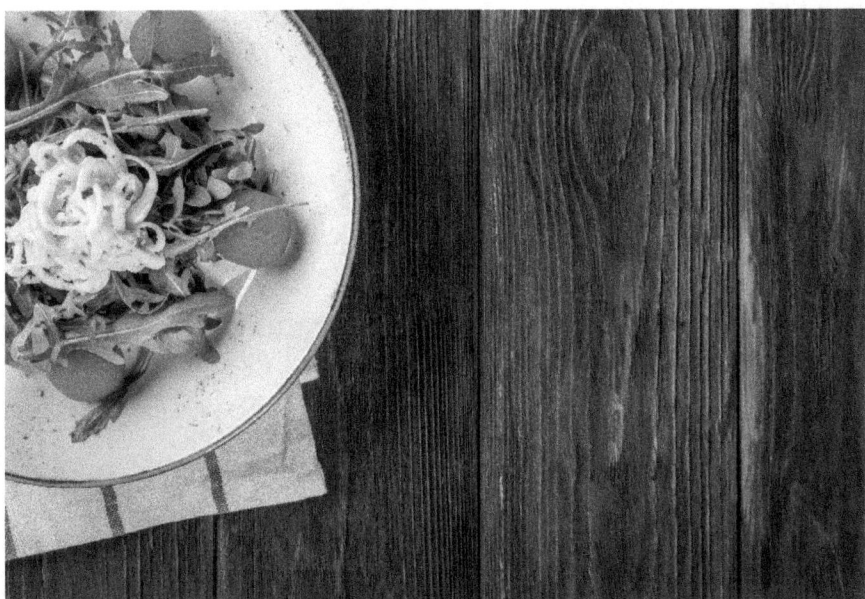

Salmon skewers

Ingredients:

2 points 600 g sliced salmon mushroom caps tomatoes onions green peppers a glass and a half of oil two fingers of dry white wine and pepper salt

Description:

create your own skewers by inserting in the skewer, either wooden or metal, the slices of salmon alternating with mushrooms or tomatoes. Leave the skewers in an oven dish to soak in wine and oil and leave for about 3 hours. After this time, place the skewers on a hot oven grill or on the embers of a barbecue and brush them often with the rest of the marinade.

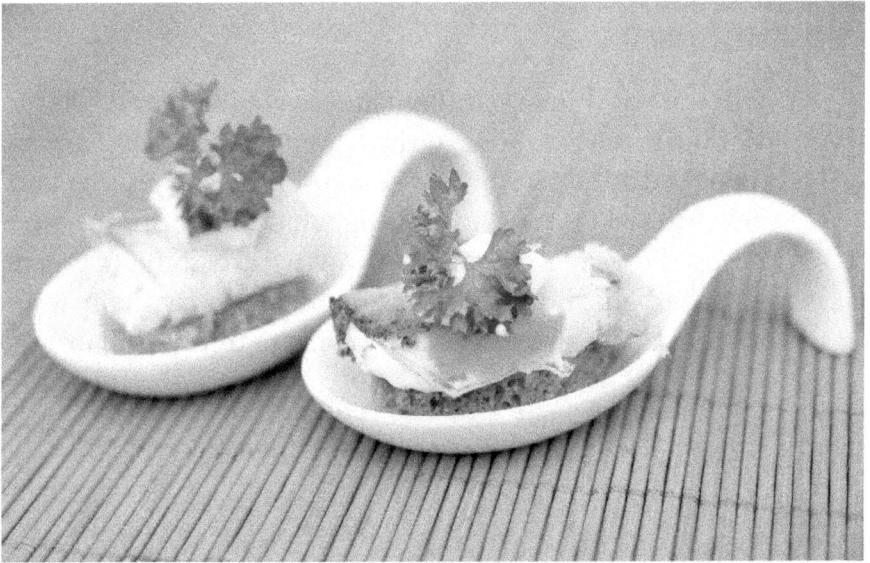

Zucchini Meatballs

Ingredients:

800g zucchini, 100 parmesan cheese, 30g breadcrumbs, thyme, 80g ricotta cheese, 1 egg, salt pepper, semolina flour, oil for frying.

Description:

Grill the zucchinis, salt them and leave them to drain for 1-2 hours in a colander, wring them out with a clean tea towel. Add the ricotta cheese, the Parmesan cheese and the chopped thyme. Add the egg and breadcrumbs, and season with salt and pepper. Now we are going to create our meatballs, flour them in semolina and fry them, then put them on a sheet of paper towels to remove all excess oil.

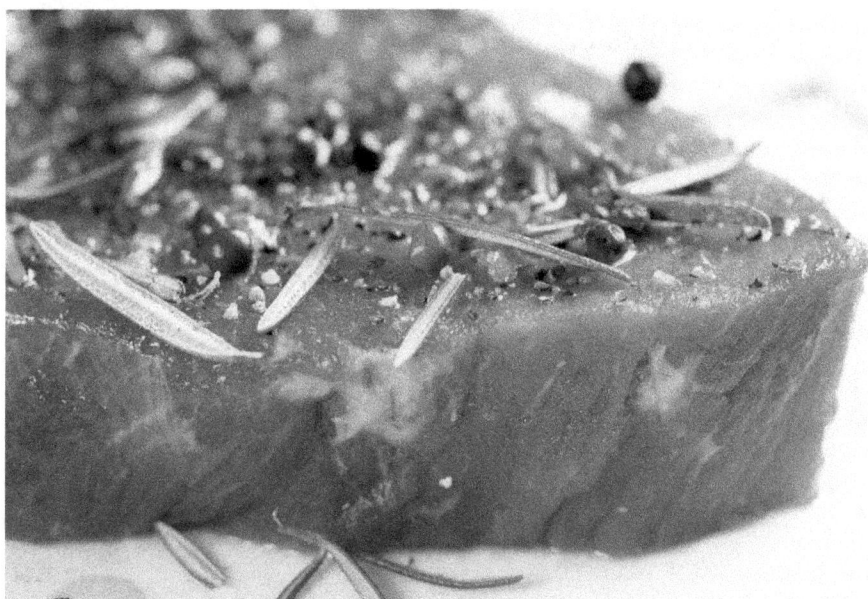

Potatoes with salmon

Ingredients:

8 small potatoes 40 g butter 100 g sliced smoked salmon

Description:

washed potatoes remove the peel and wrap inside foil to create a cartoccio but leaving the top half uncovered bake in this way at 200 ° for about an hour removed from the oven let cool the potatoes and cut them in half graphics te a small incision inserted inside the slices of smoked salmon and spread the potatoes with butter that you have melted separately serve very hot

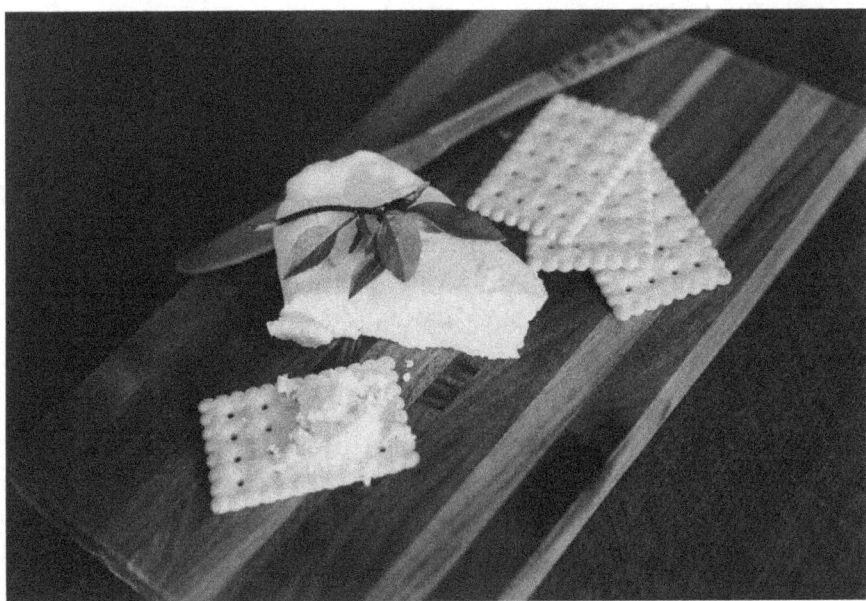

Potato Croquettes

Ingredients:

- 1kg potatoes
- 2 yolks
- Nutmeg pepper salt
- 100g parmesan cheese
- 2 whole eggs
- Breadcrumbs
- Seed oil for frying

Description:

Boil and peel the potatoes, with the help of a potato masher (or two forks) create a potato mush to which you will add the 2 egg yolks, salt and pepper, nutmeg and grated Parmesan cheese. When the mixture will be smooth, you're going to create the croquettes, you can be inspired
by the classic, or you can give the shape you want, try to stay smpre within 40 g of compound, otherwise you may have difficulty cooking. Create our croquettes, passatelel nell'uovo beaten and then in breadcrumbs, at this point we just have to
immerse them in the pan with oil at 170 degrees!

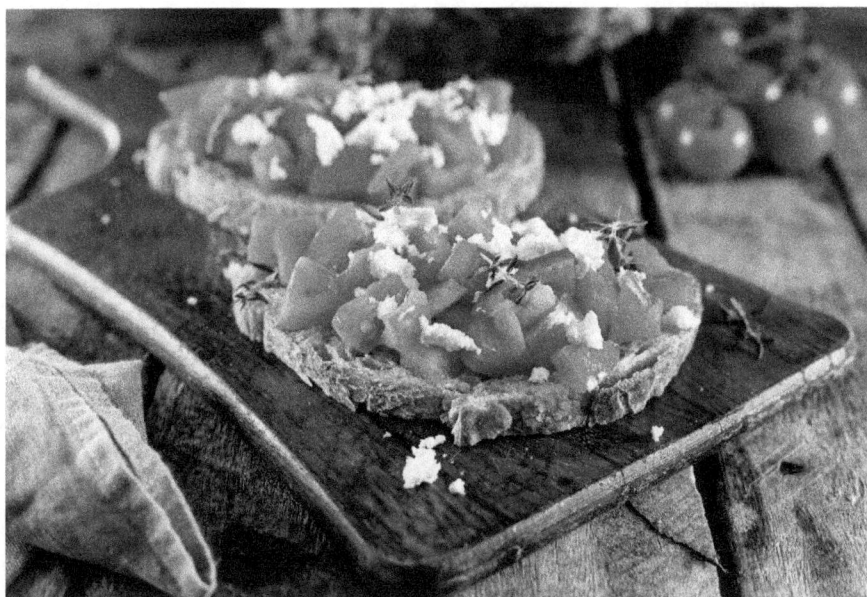

Spinach and Ricotta Meatballs

Ingredients:

- 250g spinach
- 250g ricotta cheese
- 50g parmesan cheese
- 40g breadcrumbs
- 20g oil
- Garlic salt pepper
- 1 egg

Description:

Wilt the spinach in a pan with oil and garlic, once ready add the spinach in a bowl with the ricotta cheese the parmesan salt and pepper. Add also the breadcrumbs and mix until you reach a nice smooth and homogeneous mixture; we will now go to create the meatballs, portioning the mixture, pass the meatballs in the egg and then in the breadcrumbs, I recommend cooking them in the oven 20/25 minutes at 200°, but it is also possible in a frying pan or fryer.

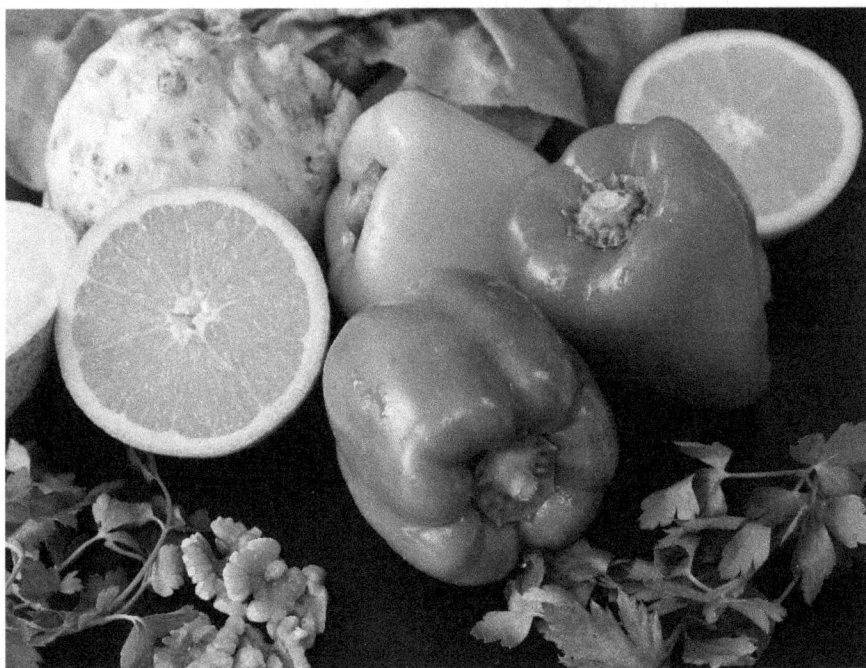

Japanese Ravioli

Ingredients:

90g Acqua calda
200g farina 00
Sle
Cipollotto cicoria aglio soia
1 tuorlo
Olio di semi
Zenzero
Tabasco

Description:

for the filling - mince with a blender, the pork the spring onion the chicory garlic an egg yolk and add also the soy sauce. Store in a covered bowl. For the dough - in the mixer put flour, salt and hot water, as soon as it is solid enough, transfer it to your work surface and knead it by hand, let it rest for half an hour in a covered bowl. Now create a coil of dough and divide it into 15 pieces, each piece will turn first into
a ball and then into a disc, on top of which you are going to place part of the filling, once closed your ravioli, you can cook them in a wok with soy sauce and hot water.

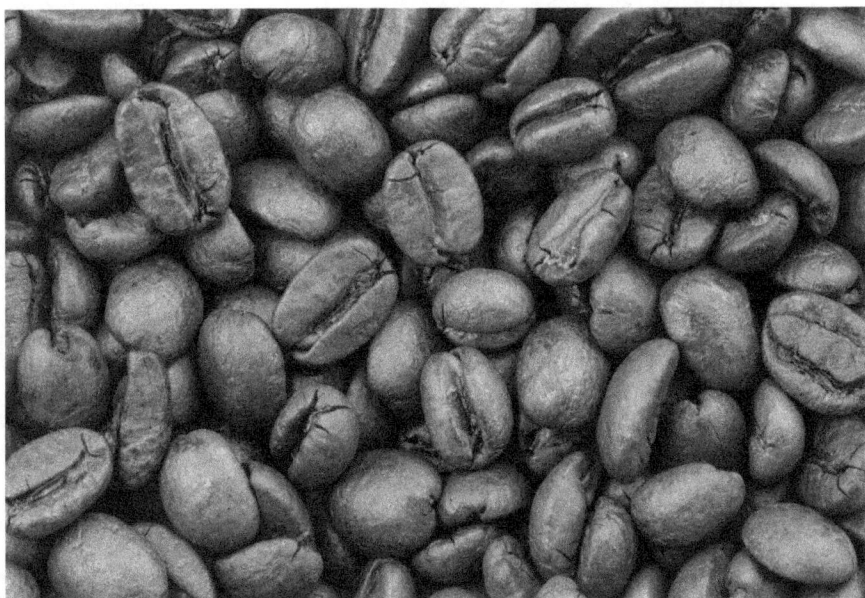

Octopus Salad

Ingredients:

- 1 kg octopus
- 1 carrot 1 celery garlic bay leaf
- pepper salt
- parsley lemon juice
- oil

Description:

Wash the octopus and remove the bag and beak and rinse under cold water, prepare a pot of carrots celery bay leaf and salt, when it is about to boil, immerse and remove the octopus 4-5 times, to curl the tentacles, at this point leave the octopus in the pot for about 1 hour. Once ready, cut the octopus into small pieces, add the juice of a lemon, chopped parsley and olive oil, leave in the refrigerator for 2 hours and it will be ready to eat.

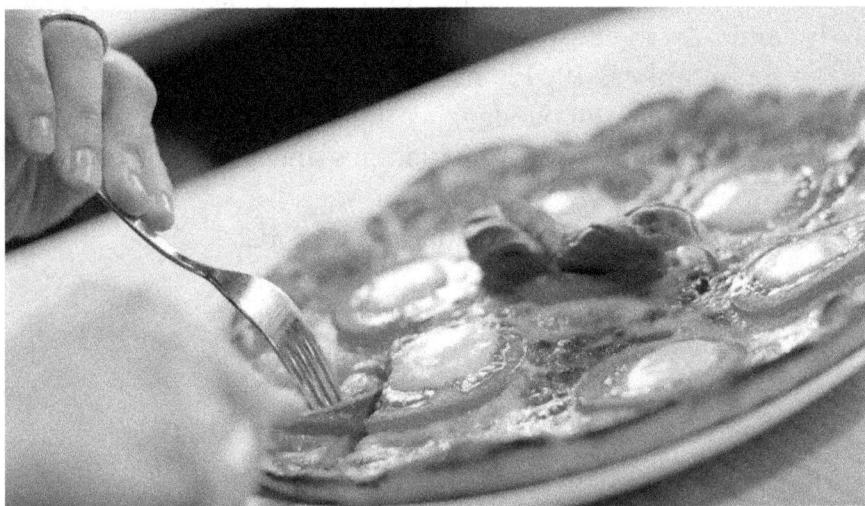

Panelle

Ingredients:

500g cec flour, 1.5l water, salt, parsley, seed oil, pepper.

Description:

cold water in a saucepan, add the flour, keep off the heat and mix, then turn on the heat, add salt and pepper, cook for another 10/15 minutes. Off the heat we can incorporate the parsley, lay the mixture in a tray and let it cool, then cut it into triangles and fry them one at a time!
The ideal is to eat it inside sesame rolls!

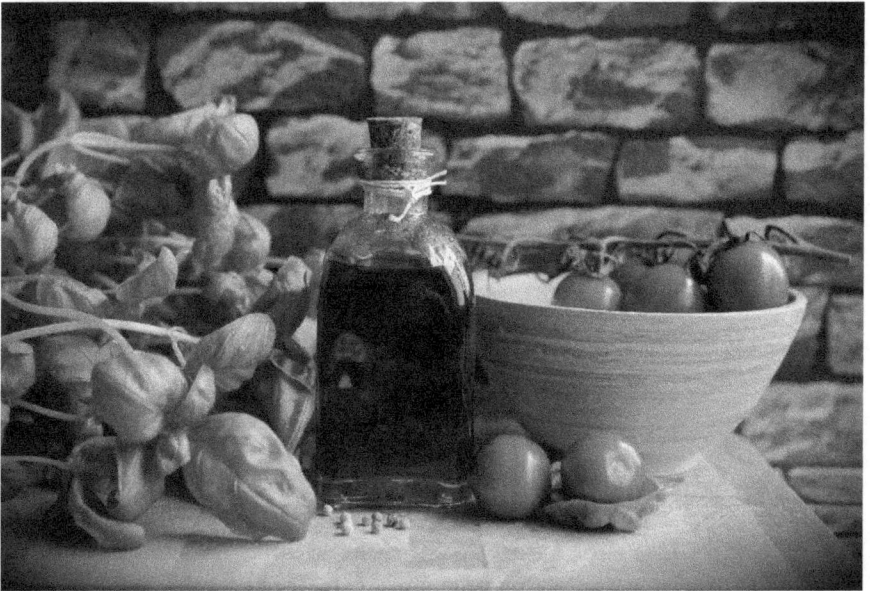

Chicken Nugget

Ingredients:

- 500g chicken
- 80g bread
- 1 onion
- mustard
- 80g flour 00
- 80g milk
- 1 egg
- Breadcrumbs

Description:

create a batter of flour eggs milk salt and mix. Leave to rest in the refrigerator. Cut the chicken and bread into large pieces, then put them in the mixer together with the onion and a tablespoon of mustard.

When the mixture is compacted, transfer it to a cutting board, where you will divide it into equal balls, which you will pass first in the batter made earlier and then in breadcrumbs. Fry at 170° until the morsels are coloured, dry with a paper towel and serve piping hot.

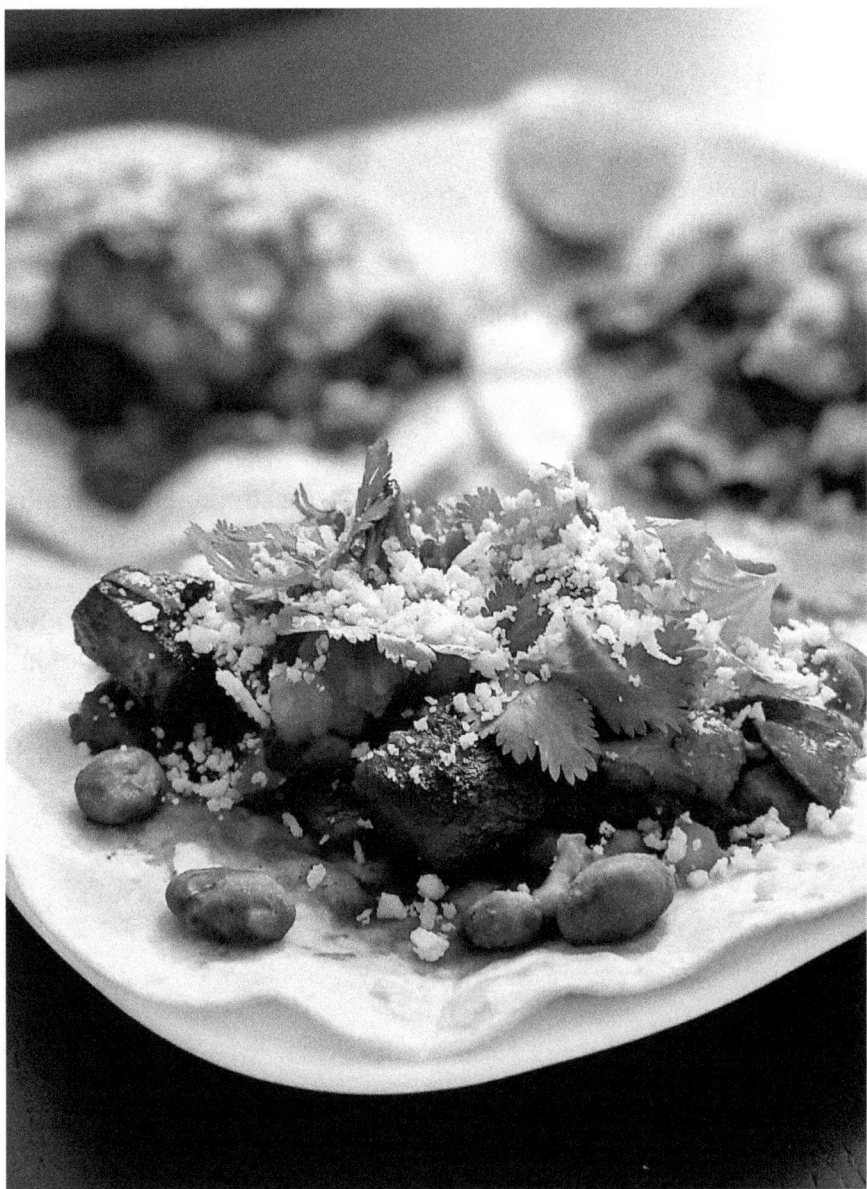

Potatoes Meatballs

Ingredients:

- 500g potatoes
- 100g caciocavallo cheese
- 80g breadcrumbs
- 60g grana cheese
- 2 eggs parsley salt and pepper

Description:

Boil, peel and mash the potatoes. Grate the caciocavallo cheese and add it to the potatoes, together with salt, pepper, breadcrumbs, parsley and the 2 eggs; now mix everything until the mixture is smooth and homogeneous. Then create your balls that will be cooked in a pan until they reach the typical golden color.

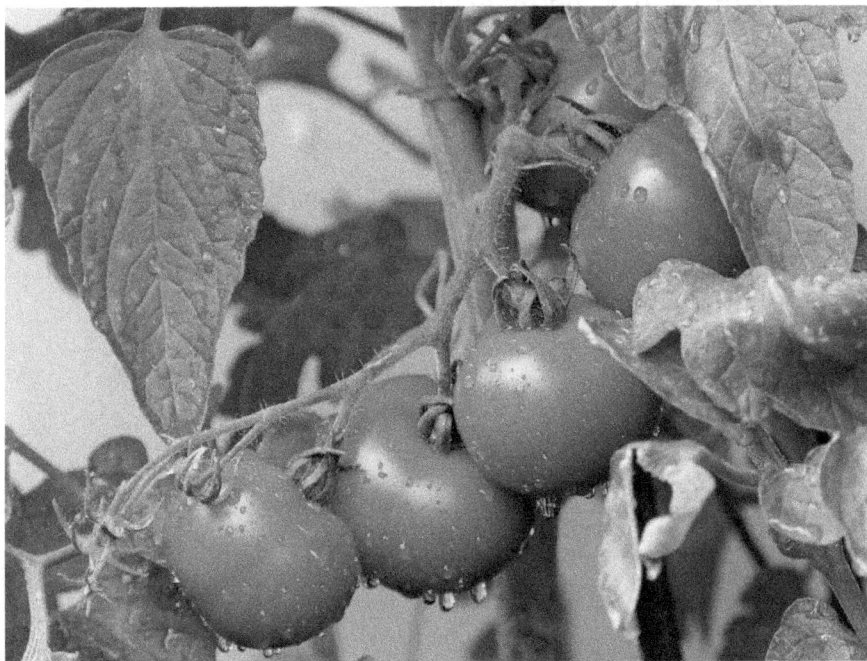

Potato Fritters

Ingredients:

- 4 big potatoes
- 2 tablespoons flour 00
- rosemary
- Salt pepper and olive oil

Description:

Wash and peel the potatoes and grate them into strips. Add rosemary flour and mix. When the oil reaches 170°, dip a spoonful of the mixture into the oil and remove it when it is golden brown.

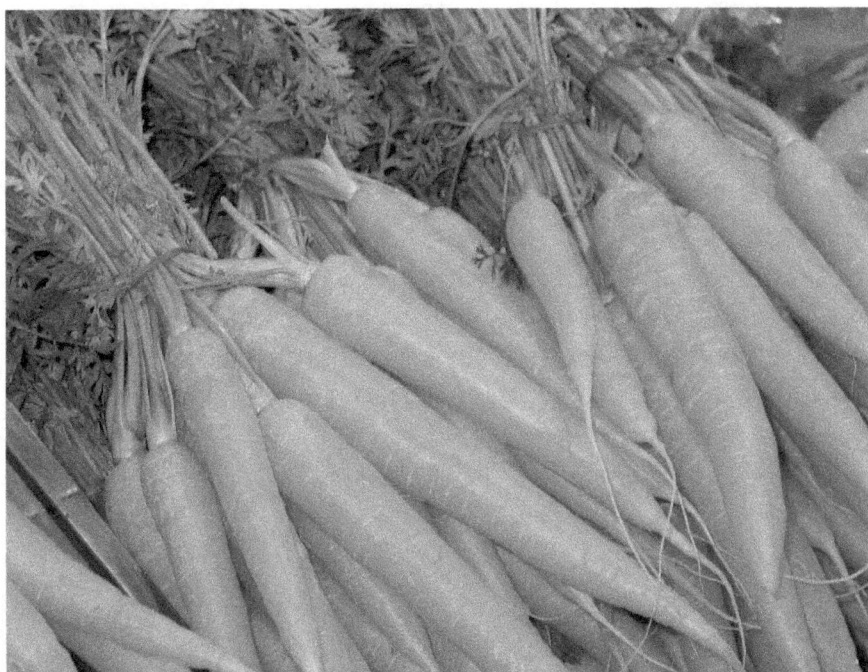

Rolled Courgettes

Ingredients:

- 2 zucchini
- 100g robiola
- 120g raw ham
- Chives black pepper salt

Description:

Wash and slice the two zucchini lengthwise, grill them on a ribbed grill pan, and put the robiola cheese in a bowl with chopped chives and salt and pepper. To compose the rolls you will have to lay a slice of zucchini, spread the seasoned robiola and lay a slice of prosciutto, brown, prepare many rolls and serve at room temperature.

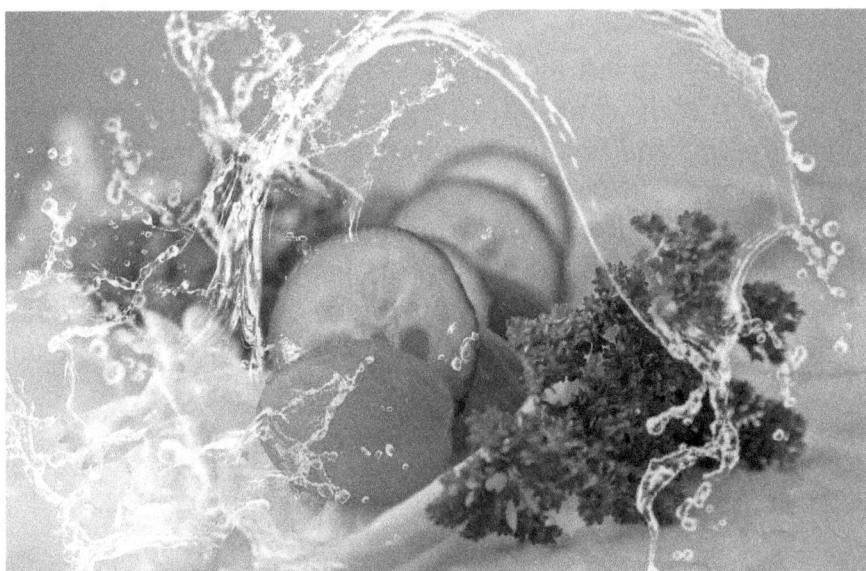

Venetian-style Bacclà

Ingredients:

500g cod, 280g oil, 1 lemon, garlic, bay leaf, salt pepper parsley

Description:

Remove the skin from the cod, cut it into slices, prepare a pot with water, bay leaves, lemon and garlic, immerse the cod and boil for 30 minutes. Eliminate the foam that emerges on the surface, then drain the fish and keep the water. Let it cool and transfer it to a planetary mixer, where you will start whirling the whisk and add the oil in a trickle, also add 100g of cooking water, when everything is amalgamated, spread it on polenta croutons and serve it.

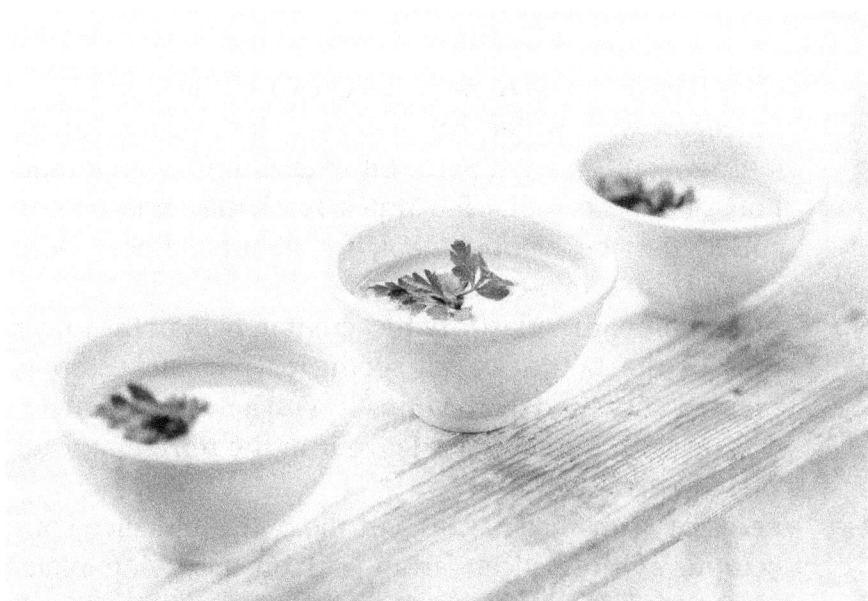

Octopus Carpaccio

Ingredients:

1.5kg octopus, 1 carrot onion juniper berries, peppercorns, celery, then lime juice, garlic, parsley.

Description:

Clean the octopus, remove the eyes and the tooth. Fill a saucepan with water, bay leaves, onion, celery, carrot, juniper, salt and pepper, boil everything, plunge and pull out the octopus 5-6 times until the tentacles are curled, let the octopus cook for about 1 hour. Once cooked, cut it in 5-6

pieces, prepare a plastic bottle, cut it in half; in the lower part of the bottle we are going to put the octopus, pressed very hard, help yourself with a meat tenderizer, close it with the peel and leave it in the refrigerator for 24-48 hours. Once the

necessary time has passed, cut the bottle and slice your octopus with a slicer, arrange it on a serving plate, accompanied by a sauce made of lemon juice, salt, oil, pepper and parsley.

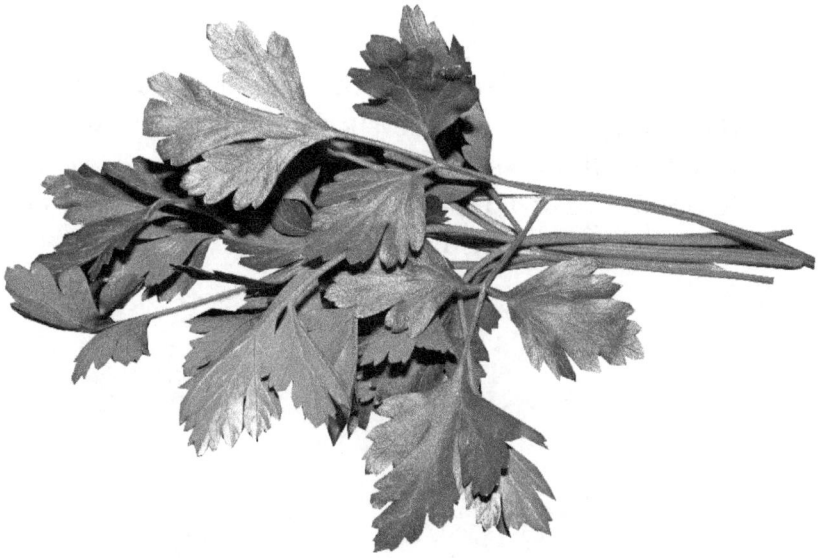

Rustic Fries

Ingredients:

- 4ptate
- Salt
- Oil

Description:

washed and peeled, with the help of a mandoline, cut them very thin, dry one slice at a time, the goal is to remove all the starch. When the oil has reached a temperature of 170 degrees, we can immerse our chips. Let's dry them once they are ready!

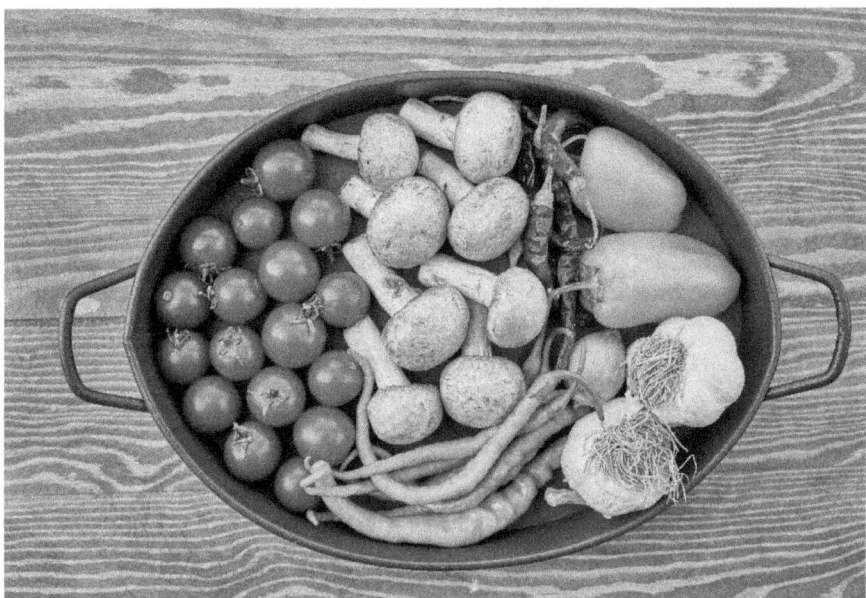

Fried Gnocco

Ingredients:

- 35g lard
- 500g flour 0
- 5g sugar
- 15g fine salt
- 125g water
- 100g milk
- 12g instant yeast
- Seed oil

Description:

Mix water, milk, flour and yeast, then add sugar and salt. Incorporate the lard and knead with your hands, then create a ball and let it rest covered for 1 hour. At this point we just have to roll out with a rolling pin our dough, and then cut it into rectangles, measures as desired. When the oil is hot fry 3 prices at a time, they should swell, dervire with slices or fresh cheese.

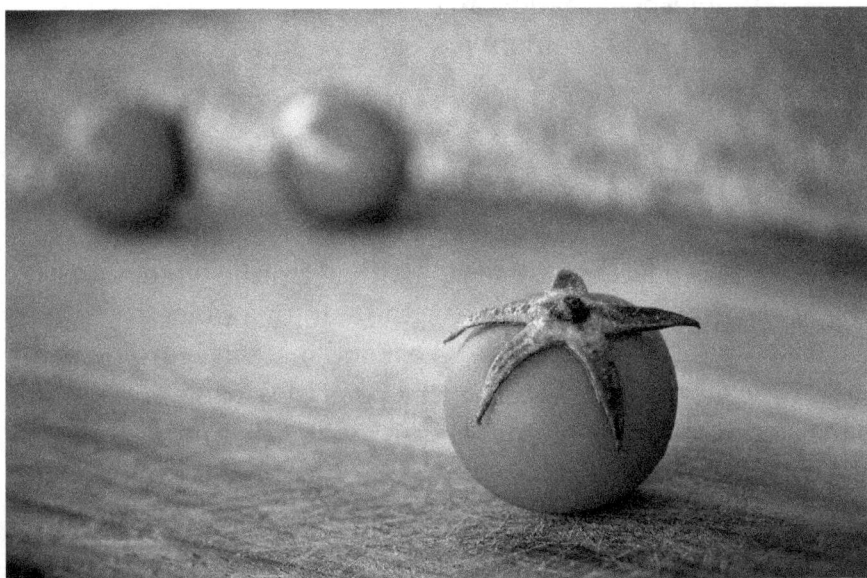

Breadsticks

Ingredients:

- 280ml water
- 155g brewer's yeast
- 8g fine salt
- 50g oil
- 1 tablespoon barley malt
- 1 tablespoon semolina
- 500g flour00

Description:

Dissolve the yeast and malt in a little water, in the remaining water, dissolve the salt, in a planetary mixer put flour and dissolved yeast and malt and turn on. Add the oil and salt water; dust a pastry board with semolina flour and transfer the mixture on it, roll out the dough to create a rectangle, let it rest until it has doubled its volume. Adremo now to form our breadsticks, cut strips from the rectangle, place them on a baking sheet and bake 20 minutes at 200 degrees.

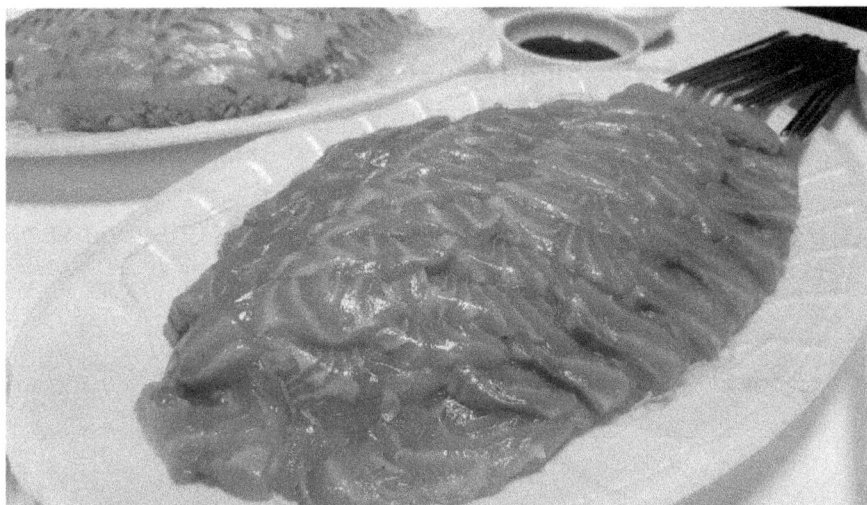

Broccoli and salmon

Ingredients:

4 slices of salmon 400 g of broccoli 1 Brico of cream 1 clove of garlic half a glass of wine 40 g of oil and salt

Description:

Clean the broccoli and create some florets cook them in boiling water for 15 minutes and then drain them in a pan put a chopped garlic together with oil and place on top the slices of salmon wet with wine and after about 15 minutes add the broccoli remove the garlic add salt, add the cream and cook for another 5 minutes over very low heat

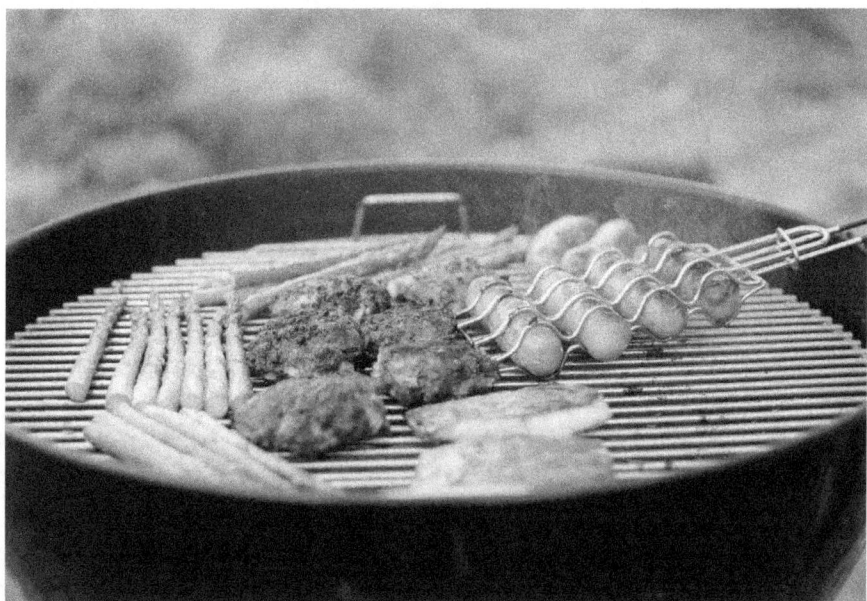

Salmon grill

sliced salmon lemon juice 60 g butter garlic parsley salt and pepper

Description:

Soften the butter, add chopped parsley and garlic, salt and pepper, put it in a cylinder or make your own cylinder out of foil and refrigerate for an hour. Heat a ribbed steak pan and place your salmon slices on it and let them cook. When the salmon is cooked, take your cylinder out of the refrigerator, discard it, cut it into rounds about an inch thick and place it on top of the hot salmon so that the butter can melt and give the salmon a shiny appearance.

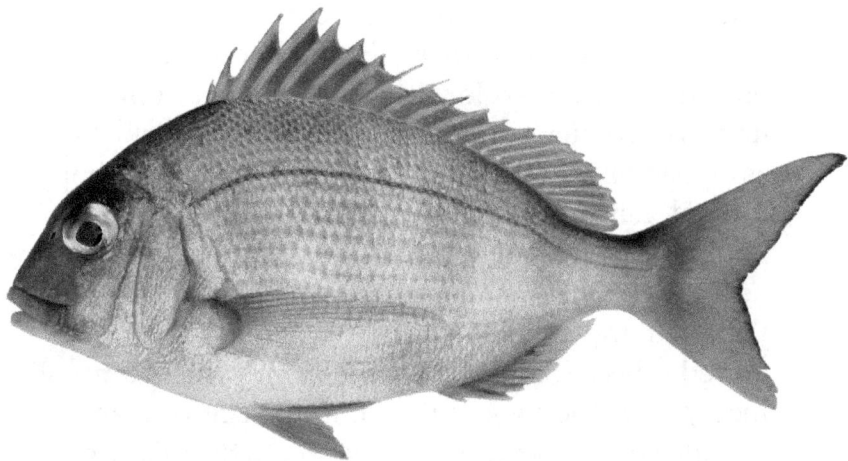

Tartine Ai Piselli

Ingredients:

8 milk buns 1 egg 40g grated Emmental 100g peas 1/2 onion 50g cooked ham 3 tbsp milk salt

Description:

Cut off the top of the milk buns, empty them of the inner crumbs and remove them. Finely chop the onion and brown it in a casserole with a non-stick bottom, turning it with a wooden spoon so that it does not stick. As soon as it begins to take color, add the milk, the chopped cooked ham and the peas without their preserving liquid. Season with a pinch of salt and cook over low heat for about 20 minutes. In the meantime, beat the egg yolk with the
grated cheese and beat the egg white until stiff. Incorporate the cooked peas into the egg yolk and after a while add the whipped egg white to the mixture. Pour the mixture into the emptied sandwiches, bake in a preheated oven at 200 °C for about 10 minutes and then serve.

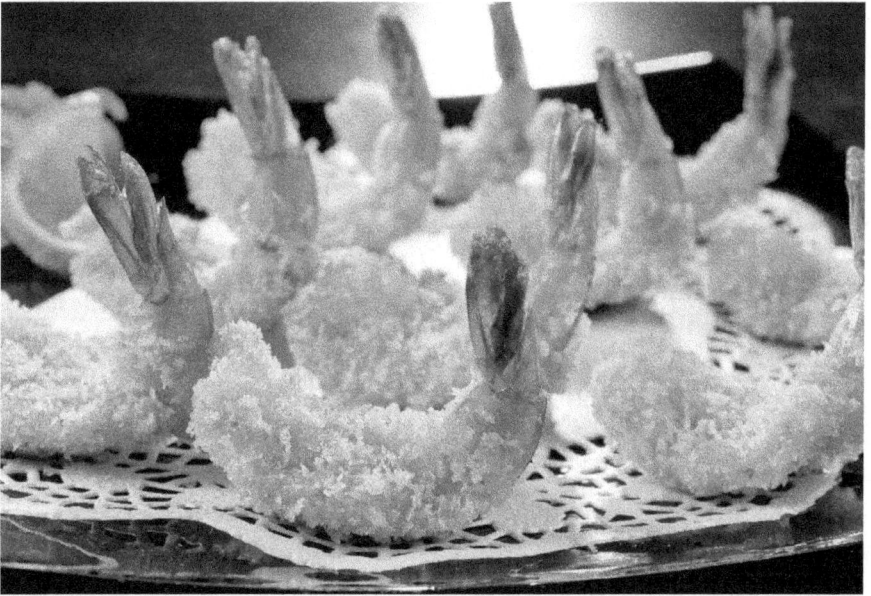

Eggplant Croutons

Ingredients:

2 eggplants 1/2 medium onion 4 tomatoes 8 slices of bacon 1 medium mozzarella Broth 1 tuft of basil Salt

Description:

Carefully wash the eggplants, remove the stalks, cut them into cubes of the most regular size possible and place them in a colander, sprinkle with salt. Let them rest for about 30 minutes and then squeeze a
little, eliminating the vegetation liquid. Thinly slice the onion and place it in a non-stick casserole with the broth, allow the cooking liquid to dry, add the eggplant and tomatoes, skinned and chopped. Continue cooking for about 30 minutes and at the end of cooking add the finely chopped basil. Cut the mozzarella into eight slices and place each one on top of a slice of bread. Divide the eggplant mixture among the croutons and bake in a hot oven at 220°C for about 10 minutes. Serve freshly baked.

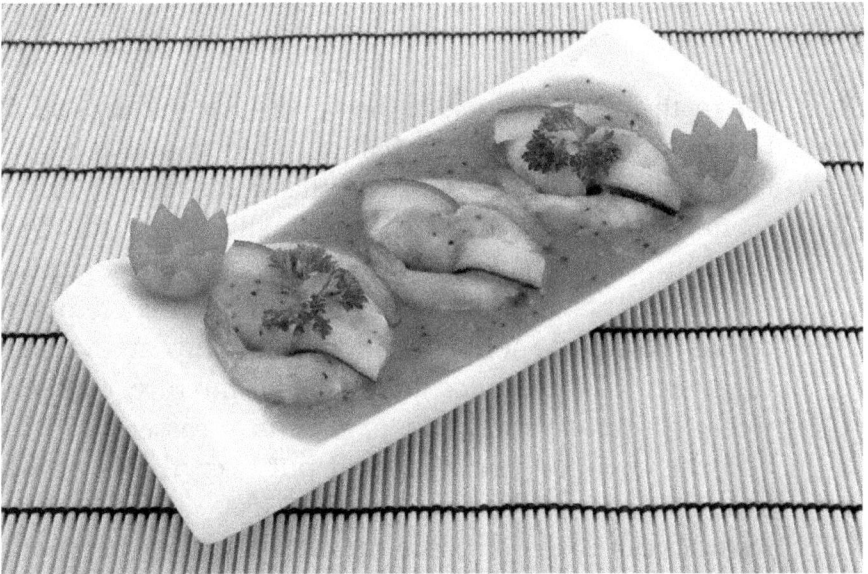

Stuffed Courgettes In Guazzetto

Ingredients:

4 zucchinis 100 g cooked ham 1 egg grated Parmesan cheese 1/2 onion parsley breadcrumbs 400 g peeled tomatoes salt and pepper

Description:

Clean the zucchini, wash them, remove the tops and bottoms and cut them in half so as to obtain 8 equal length pieces. Boil them in a little salted water; drain them and empty them using a small digger. Put the zucchini pulp in a bowl with the egg, the grated Parmesan cheese, a little salt and pepper, the chopped cooked ham and enough breadcrumbs to mix everything together. Stuff the zucchini with the mixture. Put the finely chopped onion and parsley in a casserole dish, add the chopped tomatoes and put everything on the heat. Add salt and pepper and after 15
minutes put the zucchini in the casserole dish. Let them cook for another 10 minutes and serve hot or warm according to your taste.

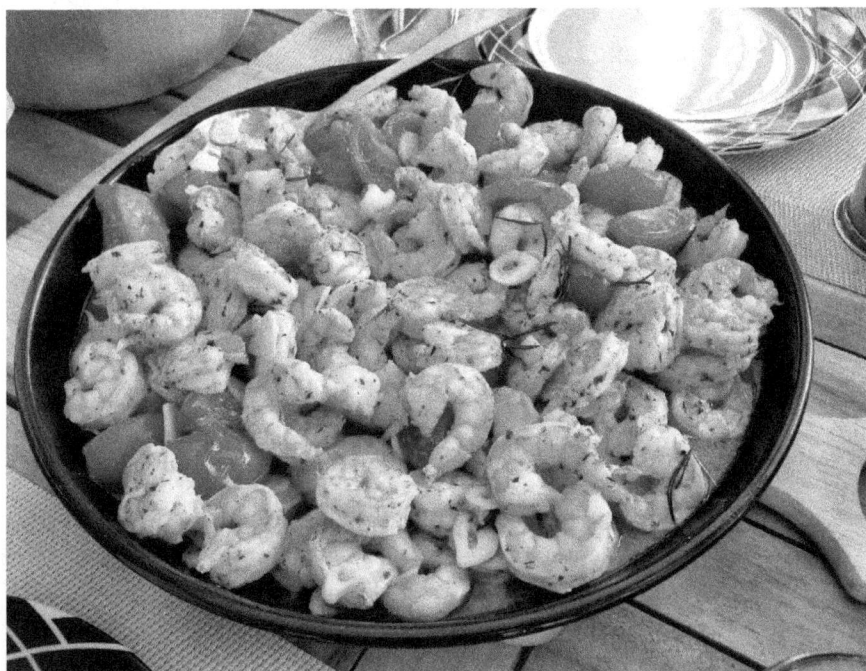

Appetizing portfolios

Ingredients:

- 4 slices of veal weighing
- 2 slices of cooked ham
- 1 hard-boiled egg
- 2 gherkins
- A whole egg breadcrumbs butter
- salt

Description:

Finely pound the slices of meat, place on each one half a slice of cooked ham, a wedge of hard-boiled egg and half a cucumber. Fold the meat in half, press the edges a little and dip the portfolios first in the beaten egg with a pinch of salt and then in the breadcrumbs. Melt a knob of butter in a frying pan and brown the portfolios on both sides. Drain the portfolios and when they are golden brown, let them cool and serve with a tasty sauce.

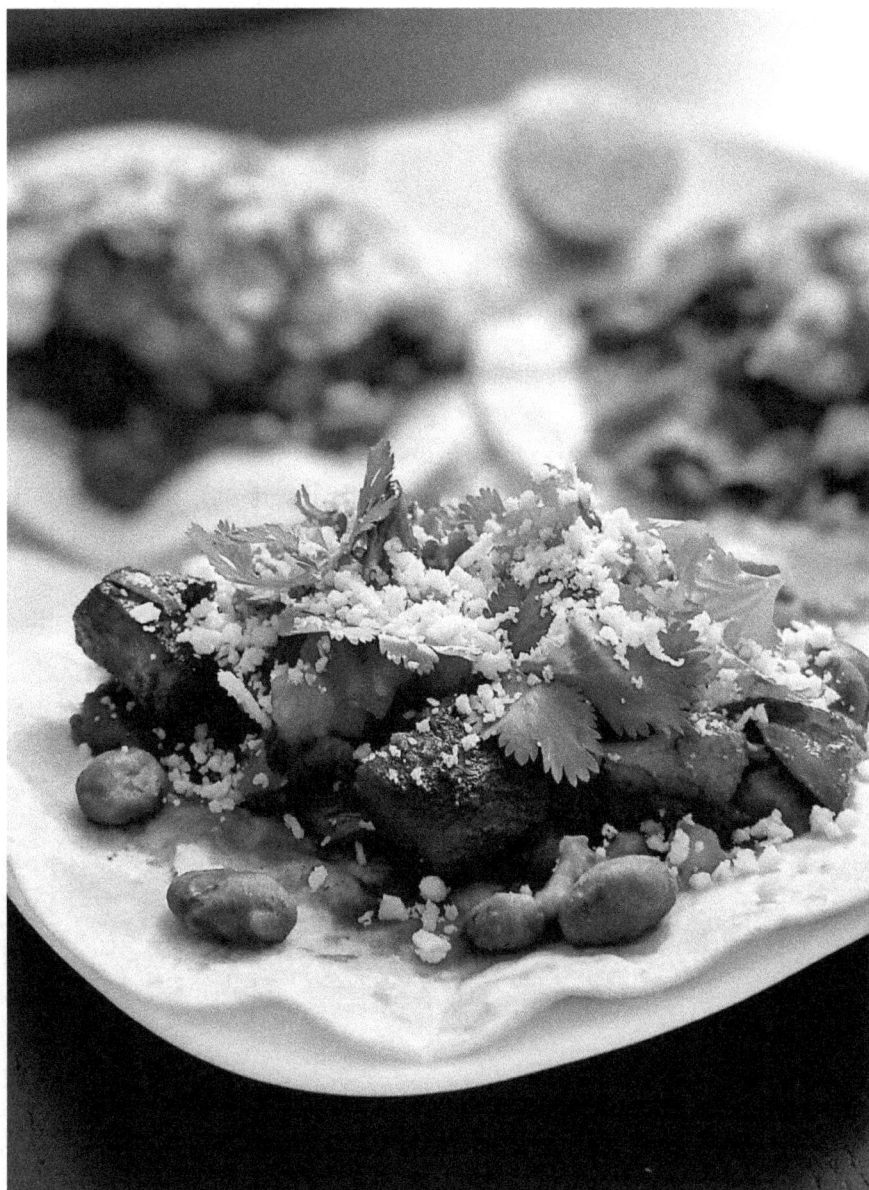

Summer Tomato Boats

Ingredients:

- 4 tomatoes
- 2 cheeses
- basil
- salt white pepper

Description:

cut and empty the tomatoes and put aside the inside cut the pulp of the tomatoes and add salt pepper and goat cheese, add also some chopped basil leaves stuff the tomato boats with the mixture serve with lettuce salad

Leeks au gratin

Ingredients:

- 1,5 kg leeks
- 1 garlic clove
- 1 ladle of broth
- 200 g of peeled tomatoes
- parsley
- 20 g of breadcrumbs
- 200 g of grated Parmesan cheese
- salt pepper

Description:

Clean the leeks and cook them in boiling water for 20/25 minutes, drain them and place them in an oven dish, mince the garlic and parsley, dice the tomatoes and place them on top of the leeks, add salt and pepper to taste, add a layer of Parmesan cheese and bake for 30 minutes in the oven. (During the last 10 minutes of cooking, turn on the grill to create a golden crust.

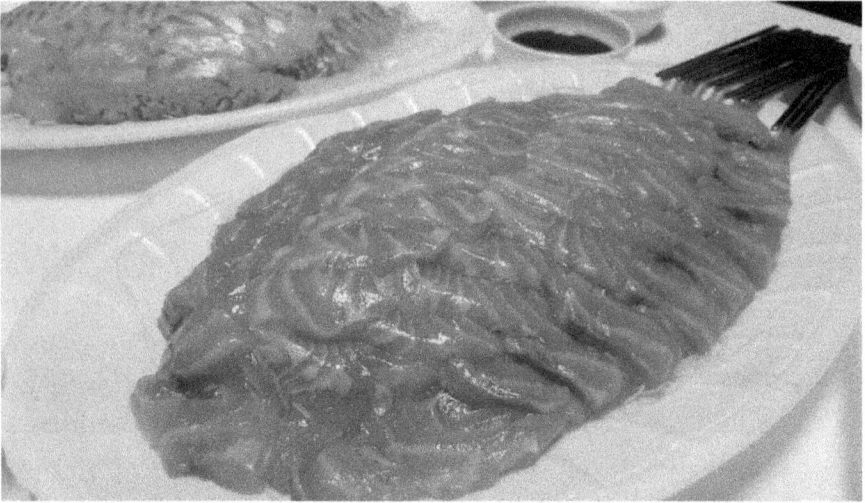

Baked Toast

Ingredients:

- bread in a box
- slices of cooked ham
- 1 mozzarella
- 1 tomato
- salt
- pepper and oregano

Description:

First, remove the crust from the slices of bread and remove any fatty parts from the slices of cooked ham, then cut the mozzarella into 8 slices and, in the same way, the tomato after washing it well and removing the stalk. On the slices of bread lay those of ham, then the mozzarella and finally the tomato, Season everything with a pinch of salt and pepper and sprinkle with a little oregano Arrange the toast on a baking sheet and bake at 180 "C for about 20 minutes or until the bread is golden and crispy and the mozzarella melted, The toast can be served as an appetizer or snack at any time of day.

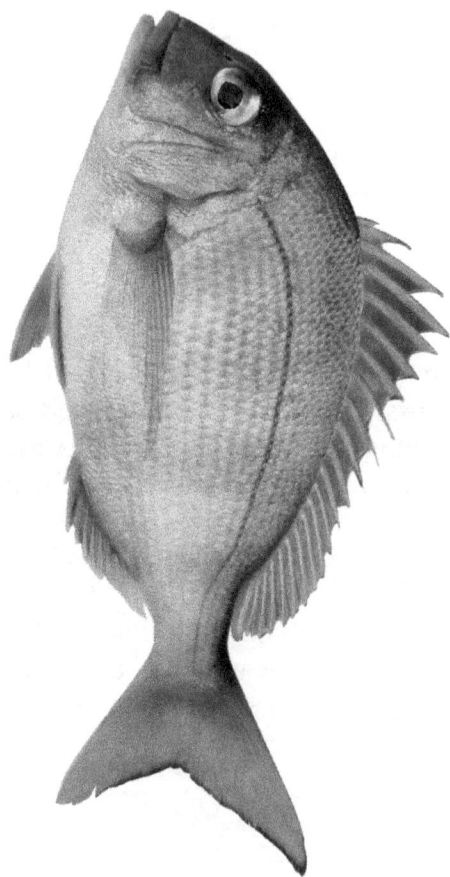

Artichokes And Golden Mozzarella

Ingredients:

- 8 artichokes
- 200 g of mozzarella
- 100 g of cooked ham
- salt
- pepper
- 1 glass of milk
- 1/2 lemon

Description:

Clean the artichokes drowned in water and lemon juice, to prevent them from oxidizing and then become dark cut the artichokes into wedges and cooked for 20 minutes in boiling water then lined with artichokes an oven dish, cover everything with slices of mozzarella, another layer of artichokes, and cover everything with ham bake for 15/20 minutes at 200 degrees serve hot

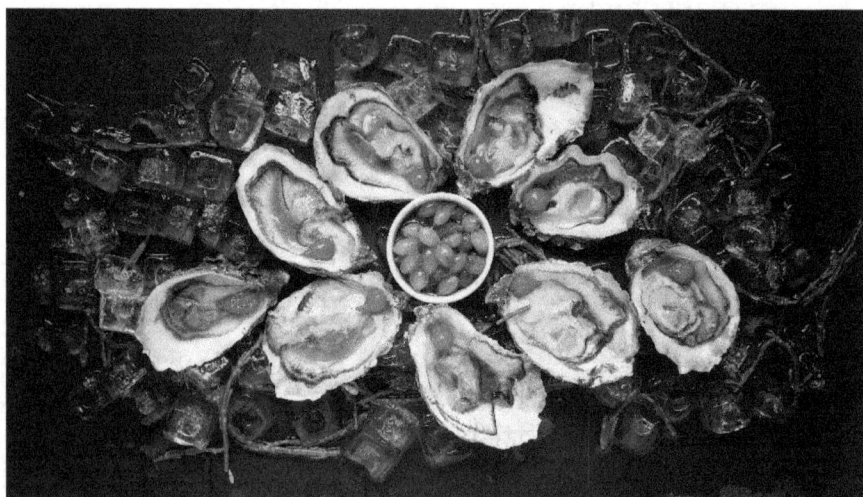

Tuna and Ricotta Meatballs

Ingredients:

- 200g tuna
- 200g ricotta cheese
- Parsley
- Breadcrumbs
- Capers
- Anchovies
- Parmesan cheese
- 2 eggs

Description:

Combine the tuna and parsley with the ricotta cheese, add the capers, anchovies and parmesan cheese, combine the two preparations and add the 2 eggs; as soon as you have obtained a smooth and homogeneous mixture, create the meatballs and pass them in the breadcrumbs. You can then fry or bake them in the oven, 200g for 25 minutes or until golden brown.

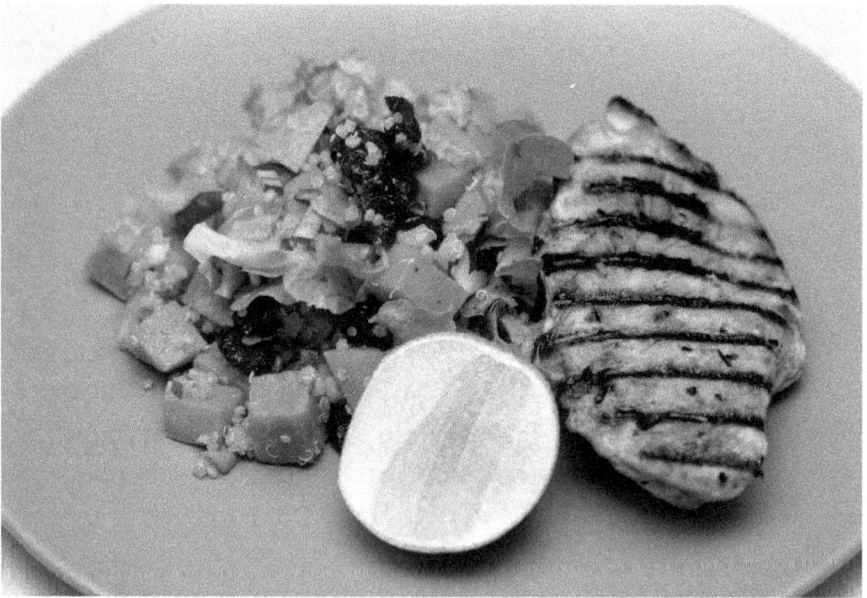

Piadina

Ingredients:

- 500g flour 00
- 170g water
- 125g lard
- 2 teaspoons of bicarbonate
- 15g of salt

Description:

Combine salt lard and baking soda, add water a little at a time and knead until smooth. Place the dough in a food storage bag and let rest 30 minutes. Then divide the dough into small balls. Lightly flour a cutting board and roll out the dough. Make circles 2-3 mm thick. In a preheated frying pan cook each piadina for 2 minutes, continuing to turn it. Fill your piadina with your favorite toppings!

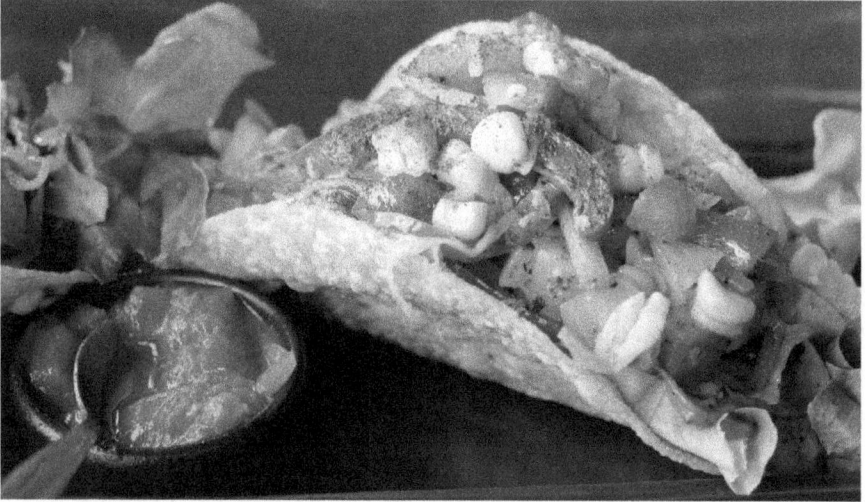

Scallops au gratin

Ingredients:

- 8 scallops
- Salt pepper
- Thyme parsley marjoram
- Oil lemon peel
- 100g bread crumbs

Description:

Put in the mixer all the spices, the oil and the breadcrumbs. Grate also the peel of half a lemon, blend. The mixture obtained will cover our scallops, which we have already placed in a baking dish ready for the fono 15 minutes at 190 degrees ventilated.

Serve freshly baked, but they are always good even when they cool.

Mozzarella In Carriage

Ingredients:

- 12 slices of toasted bread
- 500g buffalo mozzarella
- 100g flour 00
- 5 eggs
- 300g breadcrumbs

Description:

Slice the mozzarella and dry it with a clean tea towel.
Place 6 slices on a cutting board and place 2-3 slices of
mozzarella on top. Close the rolls with the 6 missing
slices and cut the rolls in half to make triangles. Dip the
triangles in beaten eggs and breadcrumbs and fry until
golden brown.
Serve piping hot

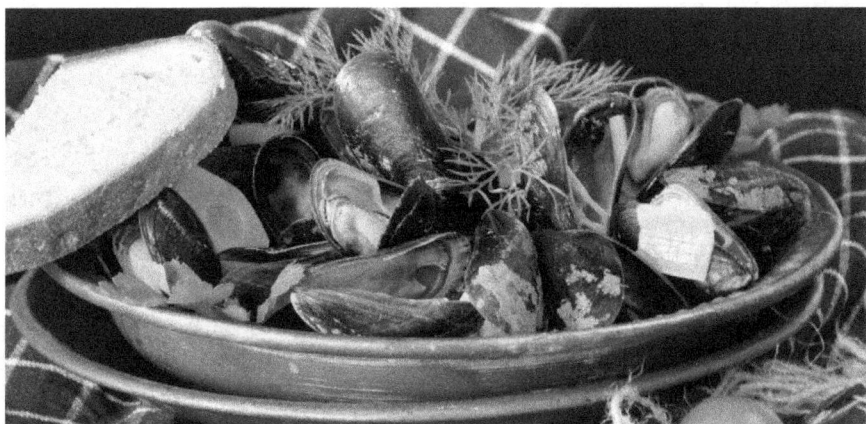

Spaghetti With Eggs And Parsley

Ingredients:

- 350 g of spaghetti
- 2 eggs
- 1/4 of onion
- 1 ladle of broth
- 1 sprig of parsley
- 30 g of grated pecorino cheese
- salt and pepper

Description:

Sauté the onions and after 3 minutes add the broth and bring to a boil. Chop the parsley and beat the eggs with a fork, add the hot broth and continue to beat.
add the chopped parsley and pecorino cheese cook the spaghetti, once drained, add them to the broth with the eggs serve with a sprinkling of parmesan cheese

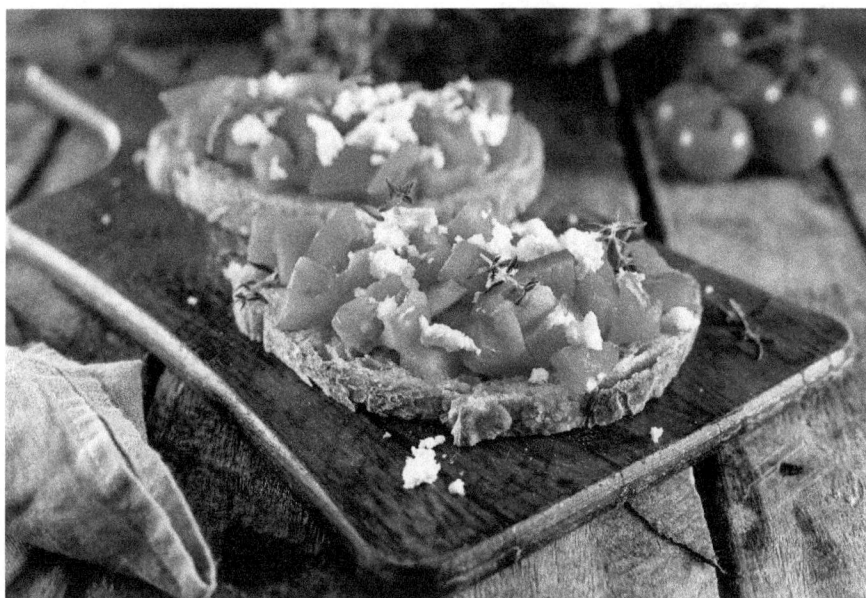

Genoese Soup

Ingredients:

- 200 g of whitebait
- 1 liter of broth
- 300 g of zucchini
- 1 egg
- 150 g of angel hair

Description:

Dice the zucchini, filter and heat the fish stock and add the zucchini, cover and leave over low heat for 30 minutes. Add the washed whitebait, pasta and egg.

Spaghetti Carbonara

Ingredients:

320g spaghetti, 150g guanciale, 6 egg yolks, 50g pecorino cheese, black pepper.

Description:

Cut the guanciale into small pieces and put it in a pan, meanwhile boil a pot of water, separately prepare the six egg yolks together with the pecorino cheese and beat them together, also add some ground pepper. When the spaghetti are cooked, transfer them directly from the pot to the pan with the guanciale, if necessary add a half ladle of cooking water. Transfer the pasta to a separate bowl and add the egg, part of which will cook, part of which will remain raw, and will give the pasta that delicious creaminess.

Serve immediately with a sprinkling of black pepper.

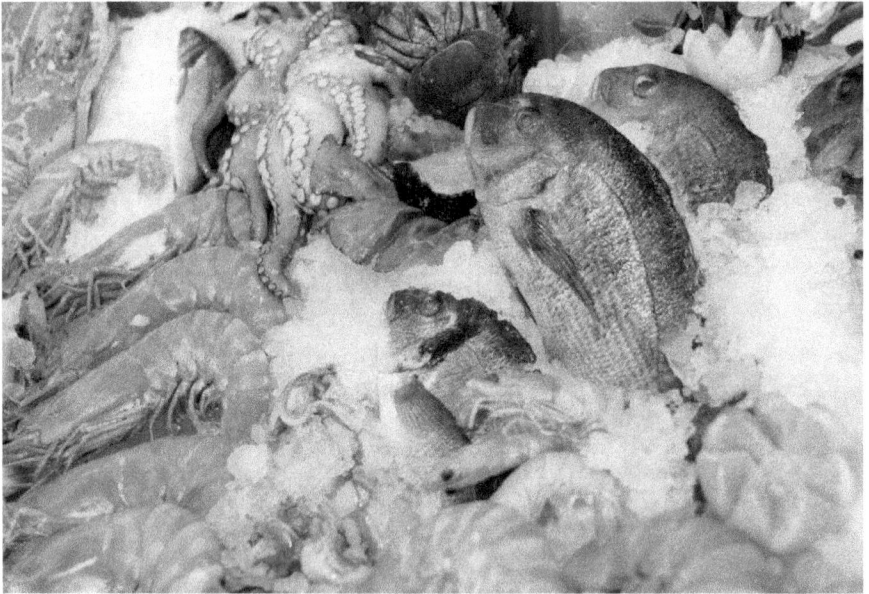

Spaghetti with Cheese and Pepper

Ingredients:

- 320g spaghetti
- Peppercorns
- Pecorino Romano cheese
- Salt

Description:

put a pot of water on the stove, coarsely pound the peppercorns and put them to toast in a pan, while the spaghetti is cooking, add a ladleful of cooking water in the pot of pepper and also add 200g of pecorino cheese, when the spaghetti is ready, I pass them from the pot directly to the pan and let mantecare, bon appetite.

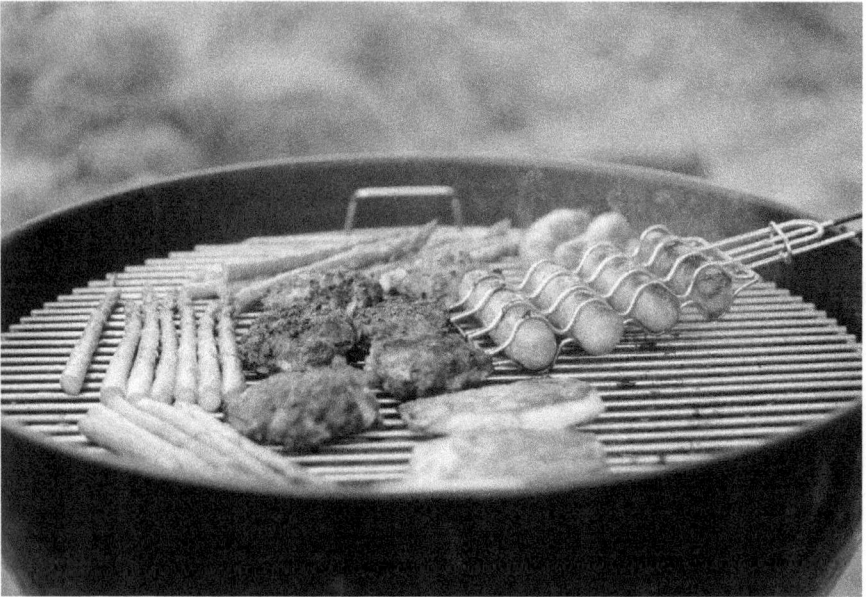

Green Agliatelle

Ingredients:

- 350 g of tagliatelle
- 500 g of fresh spinach
- 1 onion
- 1 ladle of broth
- 2 anchovy fillets
- 2 teaspoons of grated parmesan cheese
- Salt and pepper

Description:

Fry the onions cut into half moons and add the washed spinach, put the lid on and let it cook for 30 minutes. Blend the cooked spinach with Parmesan cheese and anchovies to obtain a smooth and shiny sauce, cook the tagliatelle, drain them and put them in a pan with oil and the spinach mixture and serve with grated Parmesan cheese.

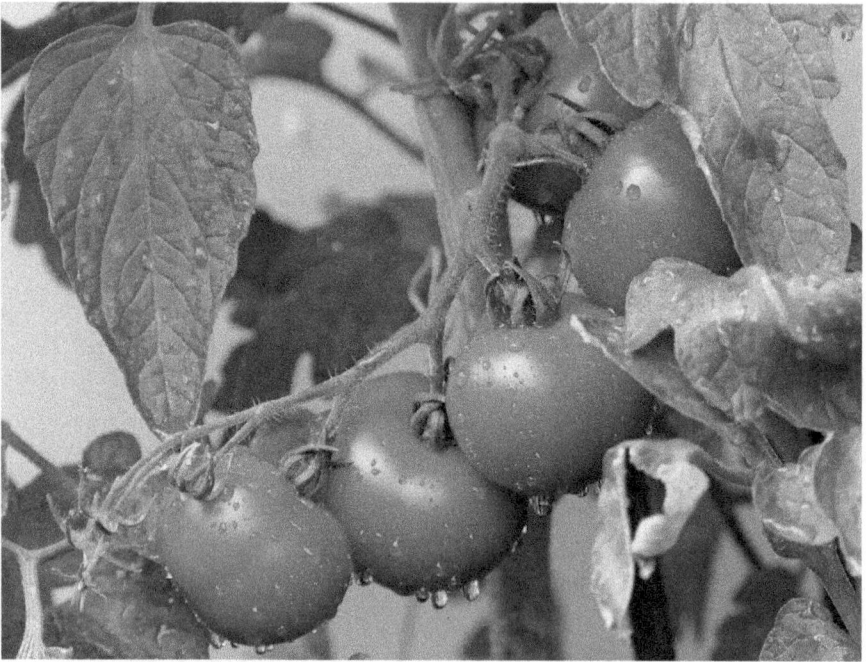

Risotto With Walnuts And Mushrooms

Ingredients:

350 g rice 1/2 onion 25 g dried mushrooms 40 g walnuts 30 g Parmesan cheese 1 liter 1/2 broth salt

Description:

soak the dried mushrooms in a bowl with water for at least 30 minutes sauté the finely chopped onion, add the rice, when it takes on a glassy color, start adding the broth, one ladle at a time (during cooking it will be necessary to add the boiling broth, the boiling will allow the starch contained in the rice to come out and create the cream) add the walnuts chopped by hand and drained mushrooms and finely chopped knife co at a time Parmesan cheese after 12/15 minutes our risotto will be cooked, add the iced butter, stir vigorously and let mantecare for 5 / 8 minutes without cover off the heat serve with a sprinkling of parmesan cheese

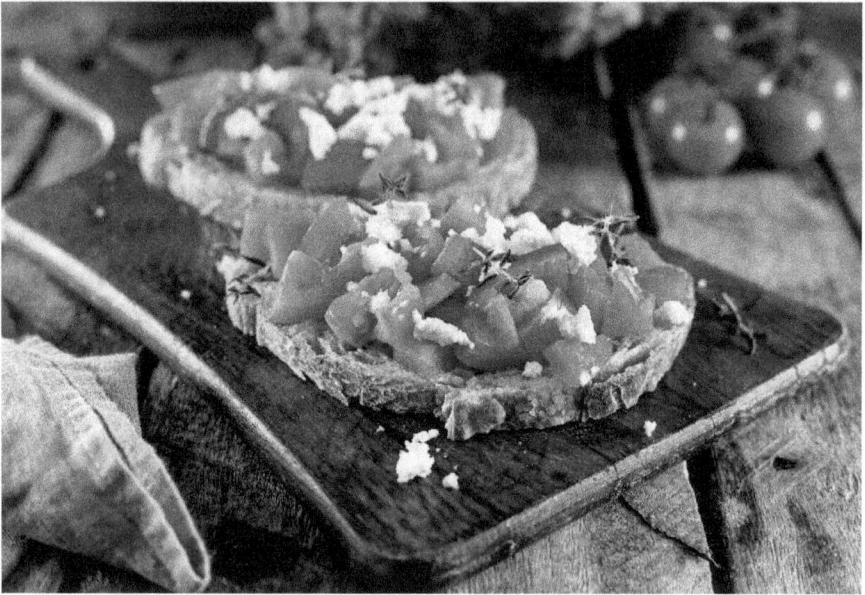

Gateau Di Patate

Ingredients:

500g potatoes, 50g salami, parmesan, 100g fiordilatte, 50g cooked ham, 2 eggs, oil, salt, pepper, breadcrumbs.

Description:

Boil the potatoes for 45 minutes, peel and mash them; cut the fiordilatte into cubes and leave to drain in a colander, cut the salami and ham into datini. Add the eggs to the potatoes, add pepper, oil and Parmesan cheese. When the mixture is compact, add the salami, ham and fiordilatte. Grease an oven dish and put the mixture, making it adhere to the entire surface, add the breadcrumbs and oil on the surface. Bake for 30 minutes at 180° and serve piping hot.

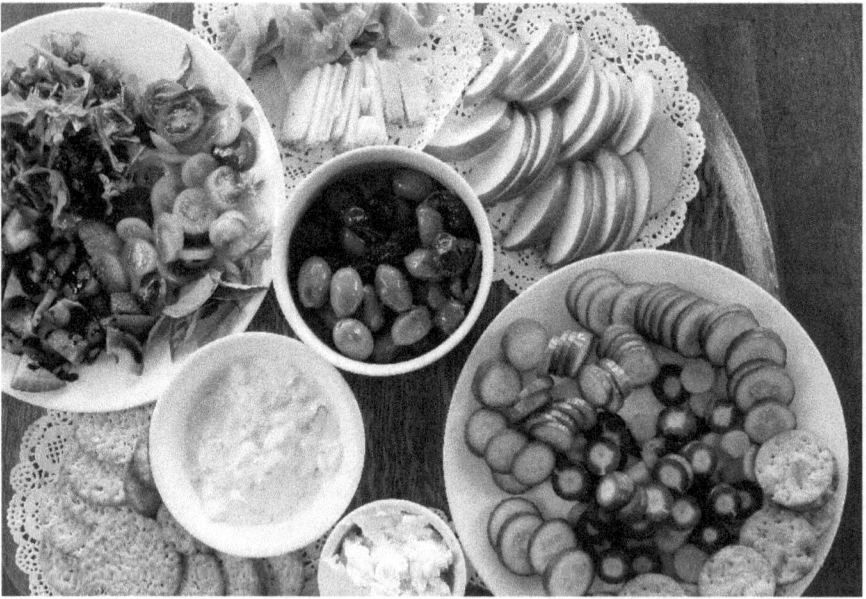

Chicken With Almonds

Ingredients:

200g chicken breast, 1 egg white, 20g water, 5g seed oil, 5g starch, 20g, almonds, bamboo shoots, soy sauce.

Description:

Dice the bamboo and the chicken, add the egg white, salt, pepper and seed oil to the chicken, add the water and the starch and mix well, cover with plastic wrap and let rest. Separately toast the almonds in a wok with unseeded oil. Boil a pot of water and add the chicken for 2-3 minutes, in another boiling water add the bamboo for 5 minutes. Assemble in a wok, stir well and drizzle with soy sauce. The best accompaniment for the almond chicken is al dente basmati rice.
Serve piping hot

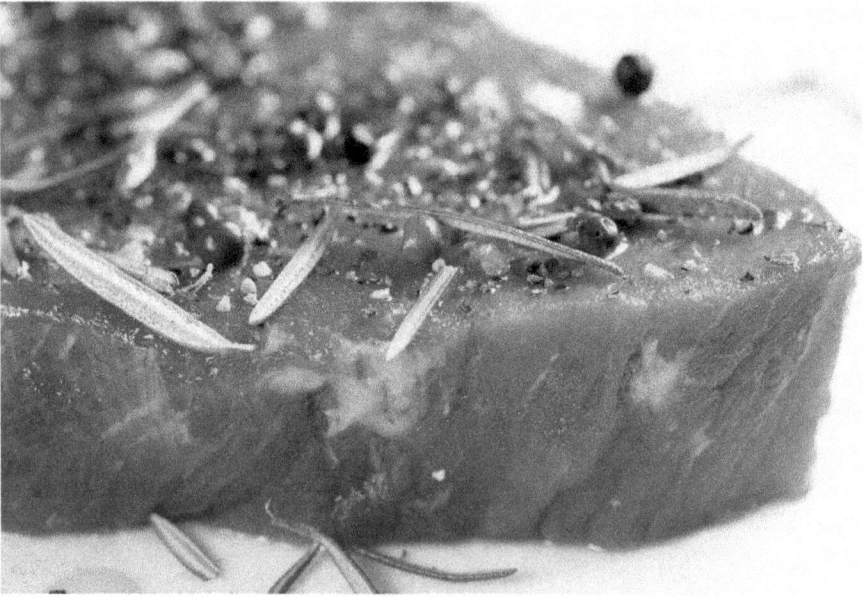

Filetot Al Pepe Verde

Ingredients:

2 beef tenderloins, 40g cream, green peppercorns, mustard, butter salt and flour.

Description:

Tie the fillet so as to make it as similar as possible to a cylinder, grease the fillets lightly and flour them ever so slightly; separately in a pan, melt the butter and put the fillets, 2 minutes per side; then add the peppercorns, lower the heat and add the mustard and cream, while cooking, with a spoon collect the sauce and pour it over the fillets. Cut off the string and serve with plenty of sauce.

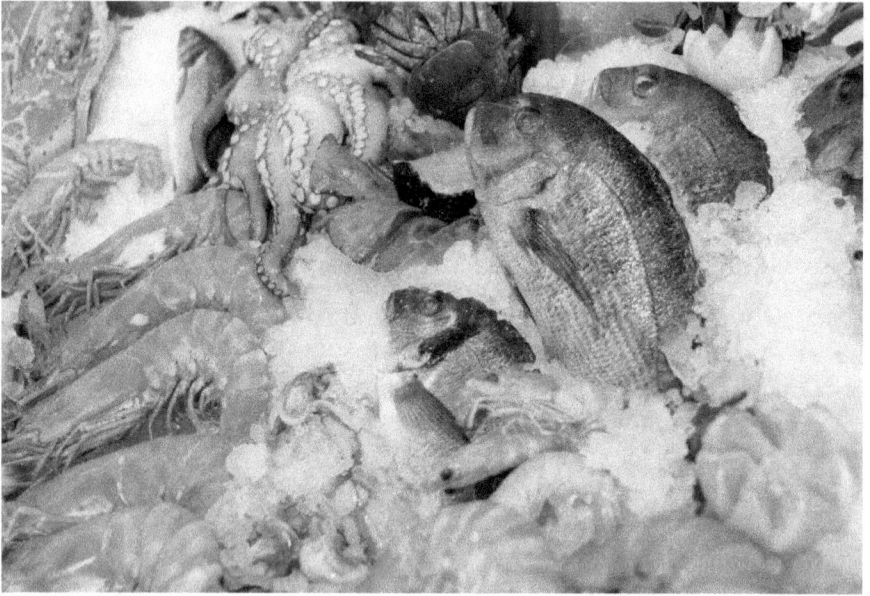

Veal Stew

Ingredients:

1 kg of veal, 1 carrot, 1 white onion, 1 liter of meat broth, 1 kg of potatoes, 1 coast of celery, oil, salt, flour 0 0, sage thyme rosemary, white wine, pepper

Description:

Chop carrots, onion, cut the veal into small pieces. In a pan, add the oil, onions and carrots, fry, and after a couple of minutes, add the veal and season with salt and pepper. 04: 05, add 50 grams of flour, add a glass of white wine and sprinkle with a ladle or two of broth, add a bunch of rosemary and cover. Separately, prepare the potatoes, peel them, cut them into large pieces and add them to the pot with the meat, add enough broth to cover the meat and potatoes, and after an hour, remove the lid and cook over high heat for 15 minutes.

Crispy Salmon

Ingredients:

1 kg of salmon fillet 100 grams of bread parsley dill rosemary thyme a lemon zest 50 grams of oil, for you in grains, salt.

Description:

in a blender insert the bread the dill the thyme the rosemary the parsley and also the hate the rind of the lemon the salt and the white pepper whisk the all take the slices of salmon remove the eventual bones, and put them on a baking sheet lined with baking paper; cover the fillets with what we have obtained free the whipped in the blender to this point we insert in the oven to 190 °C for 20 minutes around passed this time the salmon will be cooked.

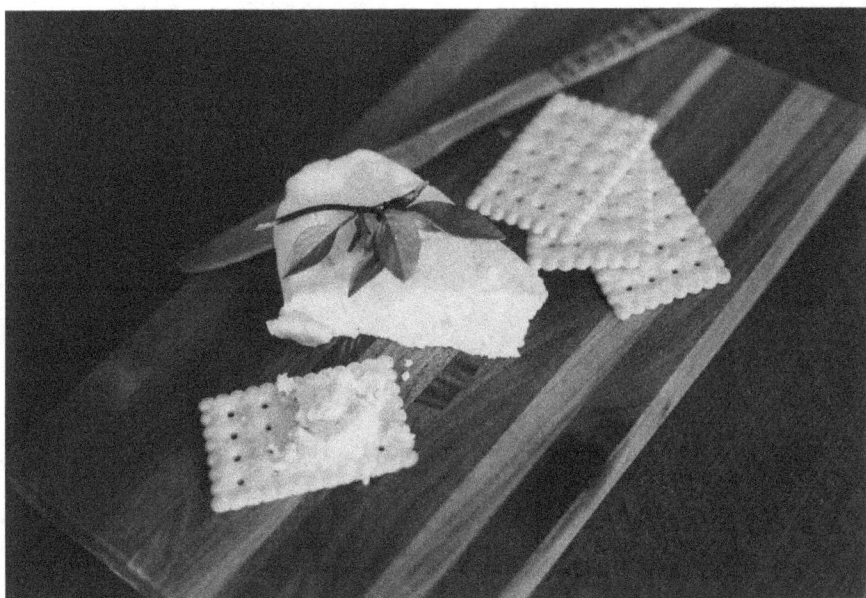

Lemon chicken

Ingredients:

600 grams of chicken breast flour extra virgin olive oil, lemons, white wine, sugar, water, cornstarch, fine salt.

Description:

Divide each breast into three finer pieces. At this point, cut strips of chicken breast from each breast, flour them, sift them and put them in a pan with a little hot oil. In a new pan, add the wine, the remaining water, the juice of a lemon and the sugar. Add the grated lemon rind, heat it up and let it melt.

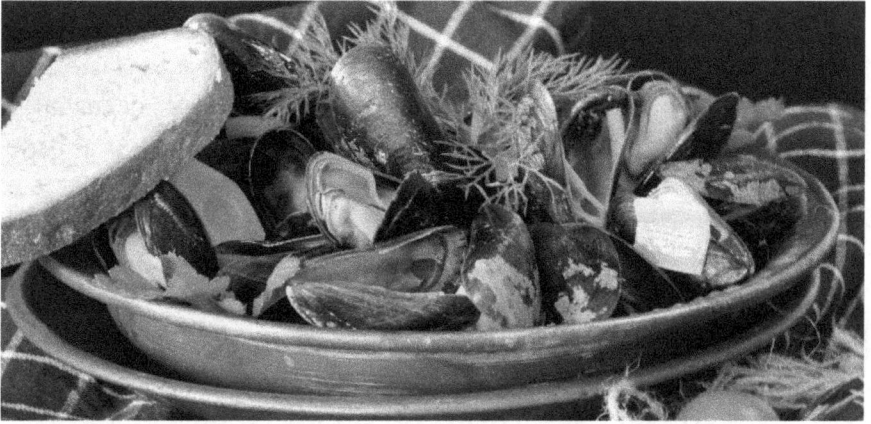

Beef stew

Ingredients:

1 kg beef 400 grams peas celery carrots flour golden onions white wine vegetable broth salt pepper oil and tomato paste.

Description:

Cut the stew into flour and place it in a pan with some oil. After a few moments, add a glass of white wine and let it evaporate, then add the chopped onions, carrot and celery and place them in the pan. At this point, it is time to add the vegetable broth and tomato paste, about a tablespoon, cover with the lid and cook for an hour and a half; after this period of time, add the shelled peas and cook for another 10-15 minutes and the stew is ready to be served at table: 15 and the stew will be ready to serve at the table.

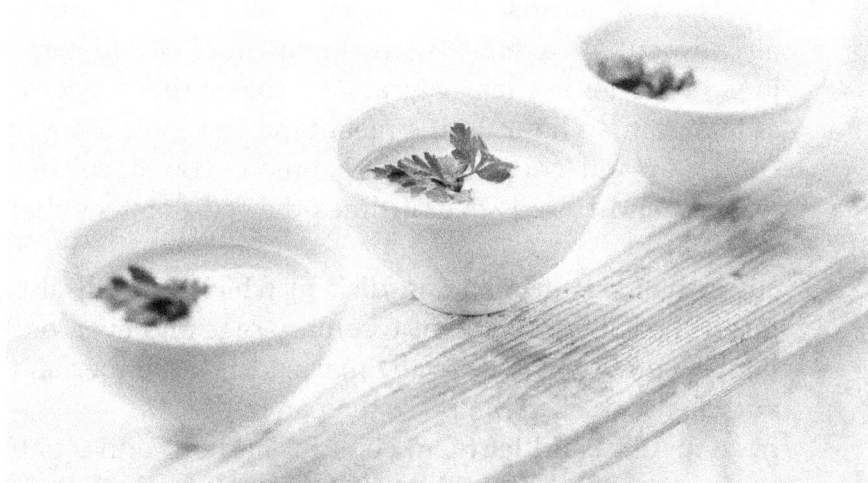

Roast lamb with potatoes

Ingredients:

1 kg lamb 1 kg red potatoes garlic water spring onion lemon juice white wine thyme sage rosemary laurel juniper black pepper salt and oil.

Description:

We create a marinade for our lamb and then we put it already cut in a bowl with lemon juice white wine juniper berries bay leaf sage and let the marinade act for at least half an hour. In the meantime you have already cut clean and chopped spring onion, you have also washed and rinsed several times the red potatoes that you will
cut in half put in a baking dish in which we will also insert the cut spring onion rosemary sage and even our lamb with all the juice of the marinade salt pepper and add plenty of olive oil; place the pan in the
oven at 195 ° and let them cook for an hour and a half two hours the result will be a tender lamb and potatoes cooked that will have taken the flavor of the marinade

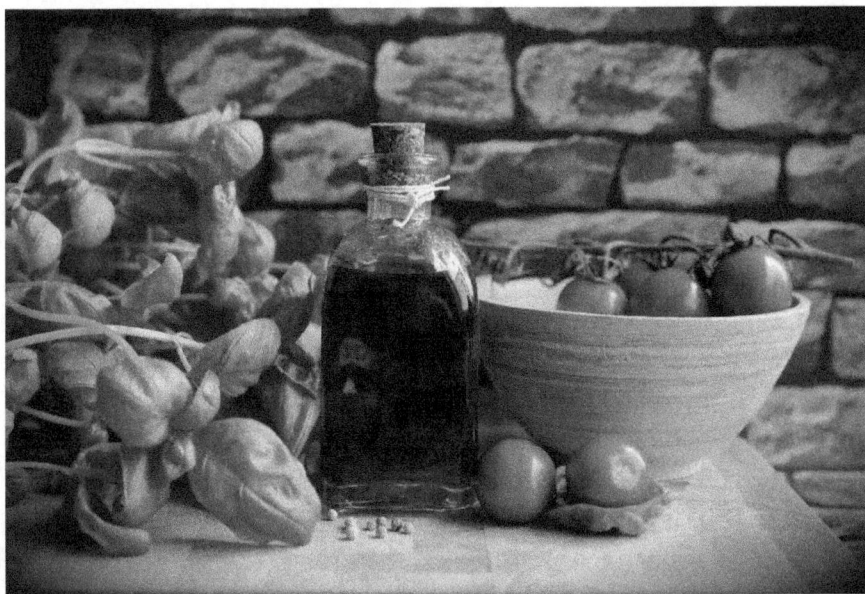

Stuffed peppers

Ingredients:

300 grams veal sausage stale bread grated Parmigiano Reggiano pecorino cheese milk eggs garlic parsley salt pepper breadcrumbs.

Description:

Cut the bread and leave it to soak in milk remove the casing from the sausage and keep it aside adding the eggs parmesan cheese pecorino cheese garlic salt pepper parsley, at this point you can also add the cubes of bread that have become soft;

when we have obtained a homogeneous mixture we could deal with the peppers cut the cap of the bell pepper remove the inside and also remove all the seeds fill with the stuffing the peppers in the top add the breadcrumbs place them now in a baking dish and cook at 180 degrees for 40

minutes after which we could give 10: 15 of grill to give them the golden color and crispness.

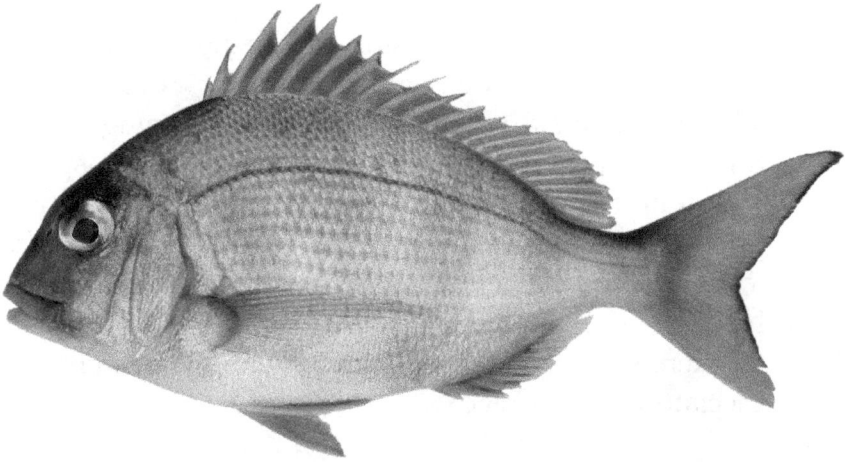

Chicken cacciatore

Ingredients:

a whole chicken 400 grams of peeled tomatoes, golden onions, carrot, garlic, celery, red wine, extra virgin olive oil, rosemary salt, parsley black pepper.

Description:

Chop the onion and set it aside, divide the whole chicken into thighs, upper thighs and breasts, put it in a pot with a little oil and start to cook the chicken, turning it from time to time; after 15 minutes add all the spices, including the ones we have previously chopped, add a glass of red wine and when it has faded, add the peeled tomatoes. Cook the chicken in this manner for half an hour or 40 minutes depending on the size of your chicken. Once ready, add the parsley and the chicken cacciatore will be ready.

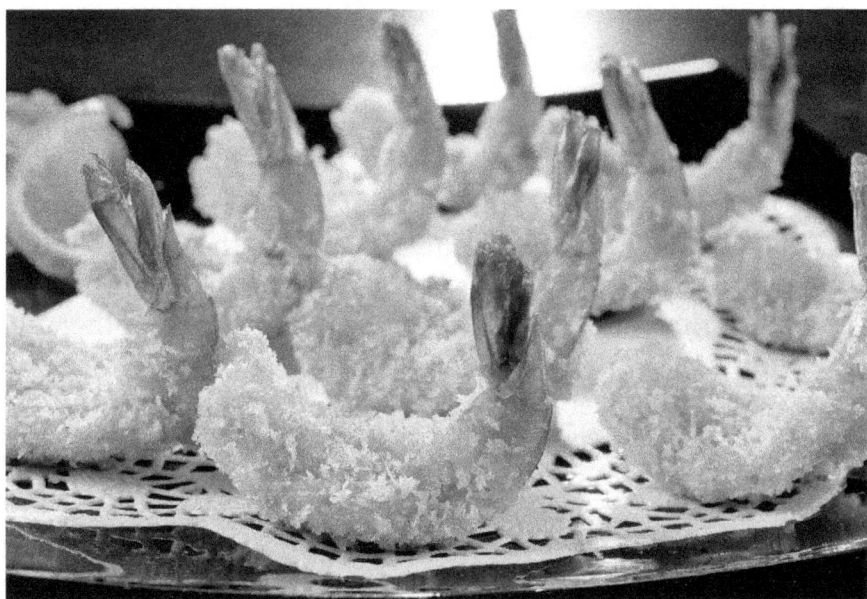

Chili

Ingredients:

800g ground beef, 250g peppers, 500g stock, 100g onions, fresh chilli, coriander, 700g black beans, 500g passata, garlic, cumin, brown sugar.

Description:

chop onion chili peppers and garlic, in a pan brown the minced meat, salt and nuance with the broth, keep the meat and in the same pan put to brown the chopped vegetables, after 10 minutes insert also the meat and the puree, salt and pepper cover with lid for 1 hour, after this time, insert the beans and let cook another 50 minutes.

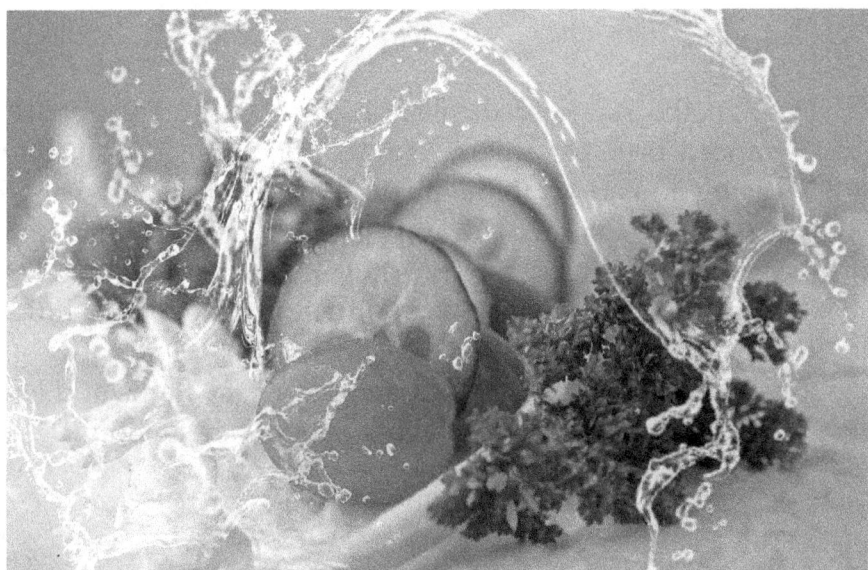

Meatballs With Sauce

Ingredients:

200g minced beef, 50g bread, 200g sausage, parmesan cheese, parsley, nutmeg, 1 egg, oregano salt pepper, tomato puree.

Description:

Chop the stale bread, place it in a bowl and add the minced beef, separately remove the sausage from the casing and add it to the mixture, place in the bowl also the Parmesan cheese, nutmeg, egg, oregano, salt and pepper. When the mixture is well amalgamated, make some meatballs, which you will put in a pan with a little oil and start to cook them on a high flame; after 4 minutes, add the tomato puree, lower the flame and let the sauce cook the meatballs for about half an hour.

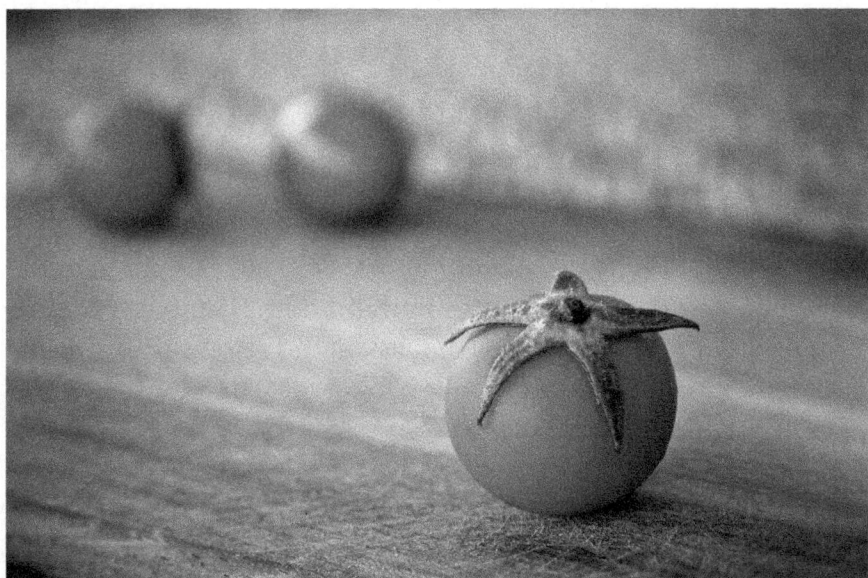

Roasted Rice

Ingredients:

350 g rice 1/2 onion 1 liter 1/2 stock 1 artichoke 200 g peas 20 g dried mushrooms 150 g peeled tomatoes 30 g grated Parmesan cheese salt and pepper

Description:

soak the dried mushrooms in a bowl with water for at least 30 minutes sauté the finely chopped onion, add the artichoke cleaned and thinly sliced add a ladle of broth let it boil 10 minutes add the drained mushrooms and chopped with a knife, tomatoes, salt and pepper to taste, let it cook for 15 minutes with lid then add the rice, after 12/15 minutes it will be cooked, add the broth during cooking if needed (during cooking it will be necessary to add the boiling broth, the boiling will allow the starch contained in the rice to come out and create the cream) arrange the risotto in an oven dish, create a layer of parmesan cheese on top and put in the oven with the grill for 10 minutes or until it creates a nice golden crust serve hot!

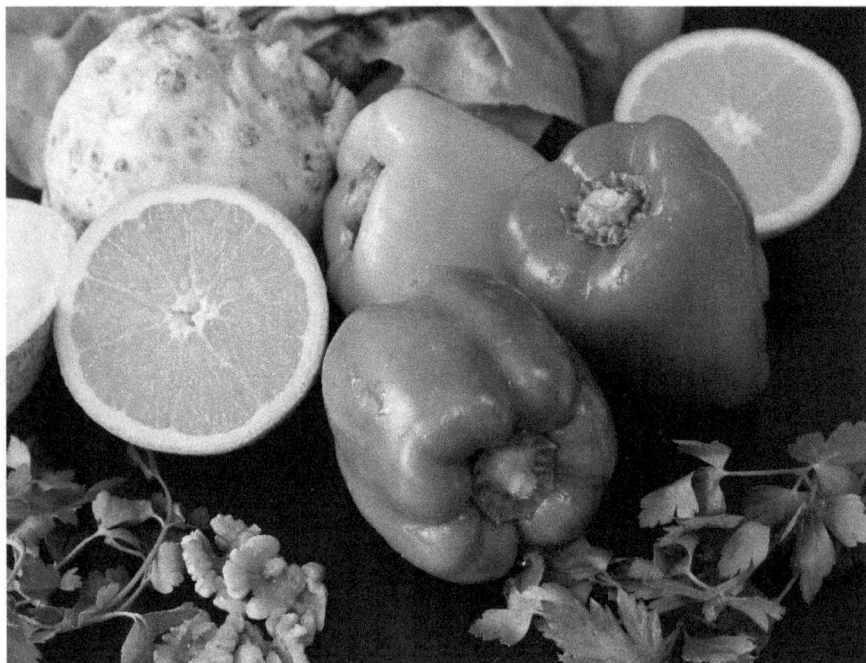

Tasty Tagliatelle

Ingredients:

- 350 g of tagliatelle
- 300 g of peeled tomatoes
- 1/2 glass of white wine
- 1 garlic clove
- 1/2 onion
- black olives
- 1 teaspoon capers
- parsley
- oregano
- nut
- salt and pepper

Description:

chop onion and fry it with a glass of white wine 4 / 5 minutes add tomatoes and cook for 20 minutes add olives capers and chopped parsley cook the noodles, once drained, add them to the sauce serve with a grind of black pepper

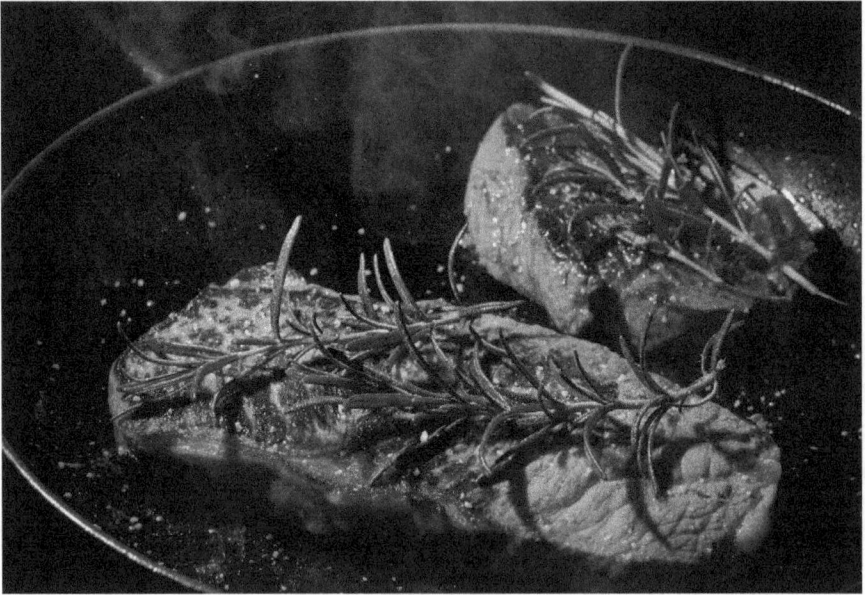

Tonned Calf

Ingredients:

800 grams of veal celery carrots onions garlic white wine 1.5l of water to their cloves peppercorns two eggs anchovies tuna capers.

Description:

Slice the carrots, celery and onion into large pieces, remove any fatty filaments from the veal and place it in a fairly large pot; in addition to the veal, place in the same pot with them two or three cloves and pepper corns, the water should cover everything in the pot, add a pinch of salt and a tablespoon of oil, turn on the heat, cover with a lid and after 40-45 minutes the meat will be cooked, drain the veal and all the vegetables, put the two eggs in a saucepan full of water until they are burnt and cut them up, put them together with all the cooked vegetables and the meat into

a glass bowl and add the desalted capers, a ladle of stock and the tuna in oil and blend with an immersion blender. slice and spread the cream over the slices of veal.

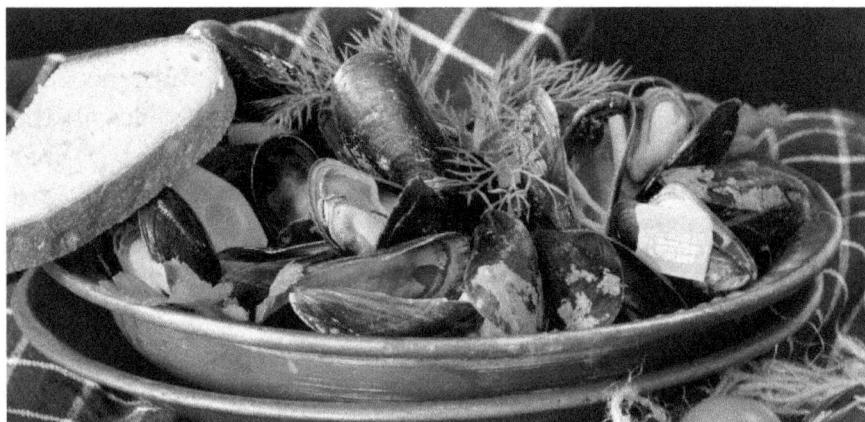

Veg – Hamburger

Ingredients:

500 grams of already cooked chickpeas two eggs 6 1 te shallot bacon fresh ginger fine salt black pepper breadcrumbs

Description:

Cut the bacon into cubes and chop the shallot aside rinse the chickpeas through a colander and then put them in a mixer with the bread, beaten eggs, mustard, add the shallot, a grated fresh ginger, salt and pepper and blend until the mixture is compact, then shape the burgers and cook them on a griddle. Ideal and eat them in a classic hamburger bun, accompanying everything with tomatoes and lettuce.

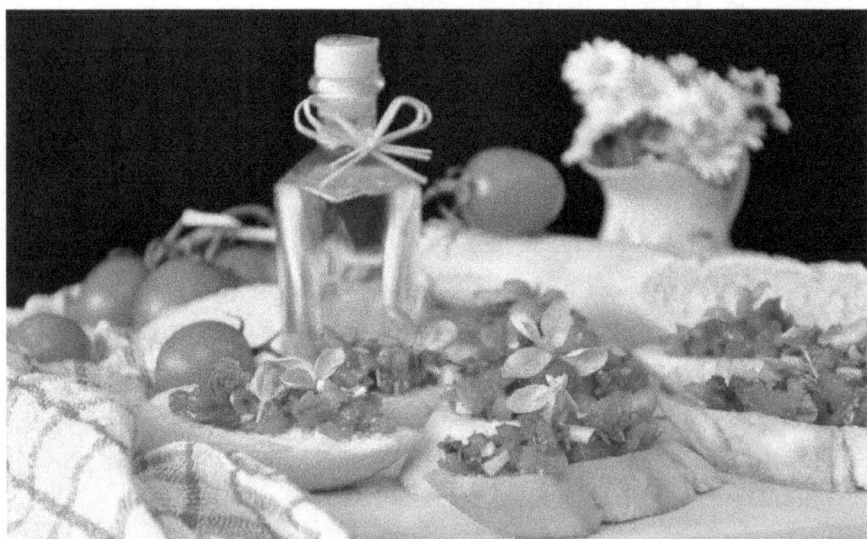

Potatoes And Sausage

Ingredients:

500 grams of sausage 500 grams of potatoes salt pepper extra virgin olive oil peeled tomatoes oregano rosemary

Description:

Create a diced potato inserted into the pan with plenty of oil salt pepper and oregano at this point cut the sausage into pieces no longer than 10 cm add them to the potatoes, add the peeled tomatoes cut coarsely with scissors rosemary and cuce proceed for 40 45 minutes at 200 ° in the oven.

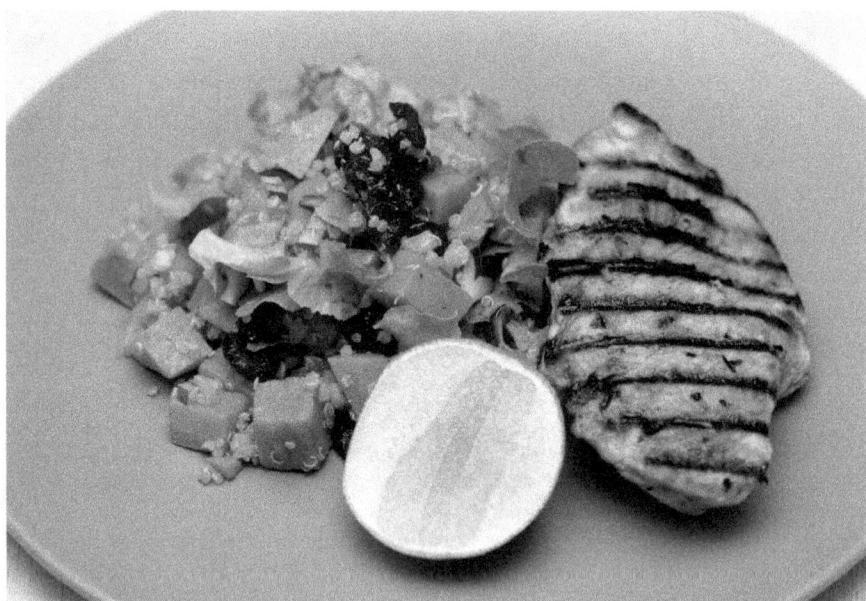

Stuffed squid

Ingredients:

100 grams squid white wine parsley garlic oil 100 grams bread crumbs anchovies parmesan cheese one egg white wine parsley pepper salt

Description:

Clean the sea rinsing several times, until you simply get pockets to fill. Separately cut the bread crumbs coarsely chopped parsley in a pan heat oil and melt the anchovy fillets to which we are going to add the garlic tentacles minced squid can now insert the bread crumbs to which we will add white wine to fade, when the pan will not be more liquid, we can transfer it into a bowl in which we will add the grated Parmesan cheese chopped parsley egg and salt and pepper. Fill our squid with the prepared mixture and chiudiamoli helping us with a toothpick then insert our stuffed
squid in the pan we used previously after 5 minutes cooked ready

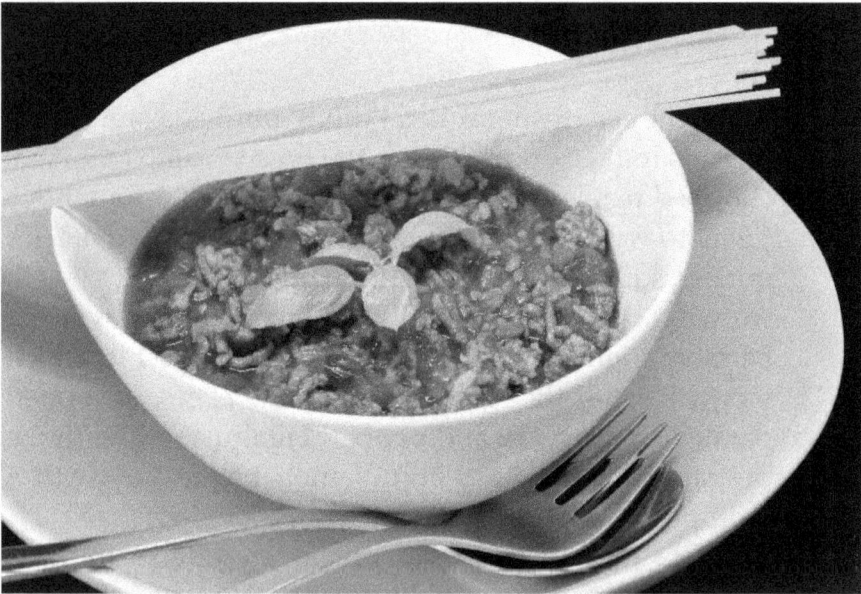

Fillet in Crust

Ingredients:

800 grams of beef tenderloin 200 grams of prosciutto crudo 400 grams of mushrooms garlic oil 20 grams of butter one yolk fresh cream black pepper salt and brisè pastry

Description:

first we will brown the fillet in a pan and let it rest in the meantime we slice the mushrooms and put them together with butter in a pan when they are cooked we will transfer them in a mixer, when the cream of mushrooms will be cold will cover the entire fillet, at this point we will place the slices of ham on a pastry board leaning diletto already covered by mushrooms in the center and we will support it with all the slices of ham, we roll
out the pastry and repeat the operation at this point we will have our fillet covered with a cream of mushrooms then ham and finally the pastry 30 35 minutes at 190 ° in a static oven and our fillet crust will be ready to be eaten.

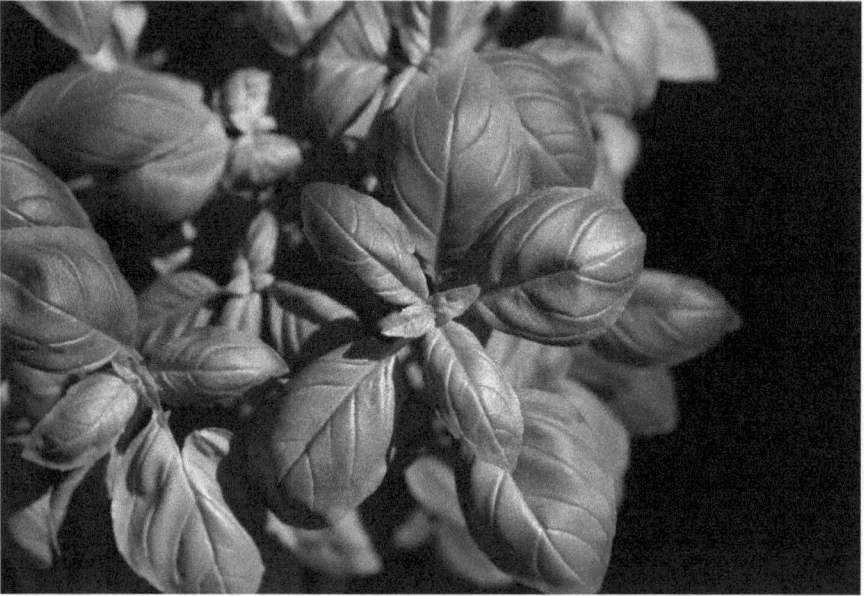

Baked sea bream

Ingredients:

450 grams of sea bream garlic black pepper thyme oil and a slice of lemon

Description:

Let's carefully clean the gilthead bream and the spring viscera completely and let's rinse it several times under cold running water. Apart from that, let's chop the parsley and set it aside; inside the belly of our gilthead we will add salt, pepper and an emulsion of oil, lemon and parsley, lastly we insert two halves of a clove of garlic and a slice of lemon cut in two wrap our fish first in a sheet of greaseproof paper and then in a sheet of aluminum foil insert it into a baking dish large enough and then we're going to cook for 30 minutes at 200 ° static fire. Once this time has elapsed we will discard our fish and serve it.

Liver venetian style

Ingredients:

500 grams of veal liver white sage butter pepper white wine vinegar and olive oil

Description:

Cut the onion and chopped sage in a pan melt the butter with oil, add the onion make it brown at this point add half a glass of water and chopped sage make it brown for 5 minutes, now is the time to add our livers of veal if the pan ended the liquid you can add another half glass of water, spent 05: 10 maximum comma depending on the size of your fillets, plate completely covering your fillets with the onions and sage in the pan serve piping hot.

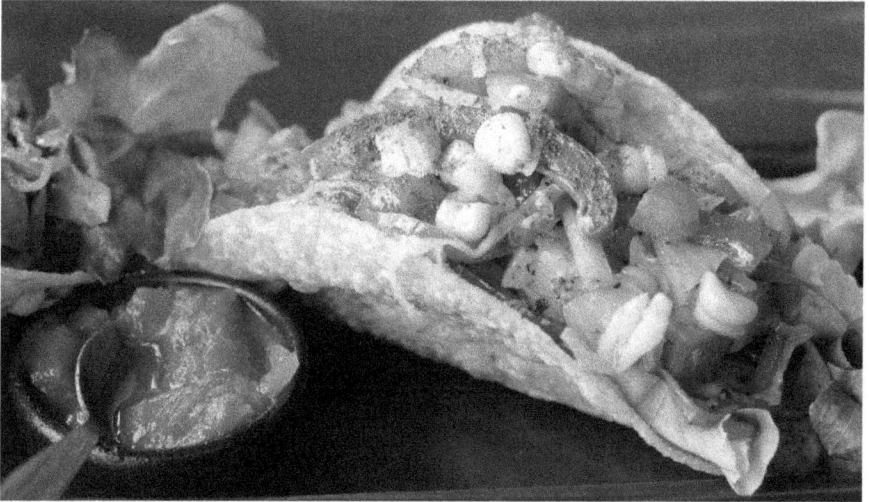

Squid in sauce

Ingredients:

1 kg squid a glass of white wine garlic oil peeled tomatoes salt parsley and black pepper.

Description:

In a frying pan add oil and garlic, when the garlic is almost burnt remove it from the pan and add the peeled tomatoes. At this point clean the squids under cold running water, once the squids are well cleaned remove the skin, when you have obtained the squid pockets cut them in half and then again in half until you obtain slices about 1 cm wide: 03 fade with a glass of white wine add the peeled tomatoes cover you let everything cook for 10 15minutes after this time add the chopped parsley. Serve hot in a soup plate.

Chicken and potatoes

Ingredients:

a whole chicken oil oregano salt sage rosemary garlic and laurel

Description:

In a blender place the rosemary, coarse salt, sage and garlic finely chopped. At this point, take our chicken and brush it with plenty of olive oil so that it becomes sticky. We are going to cover it with the chopped mixture from the mixer; place the chicken in a fairly large oven dish and bake it at 200° in a static oven for about an hour and a half, depending on the size of your chicken.

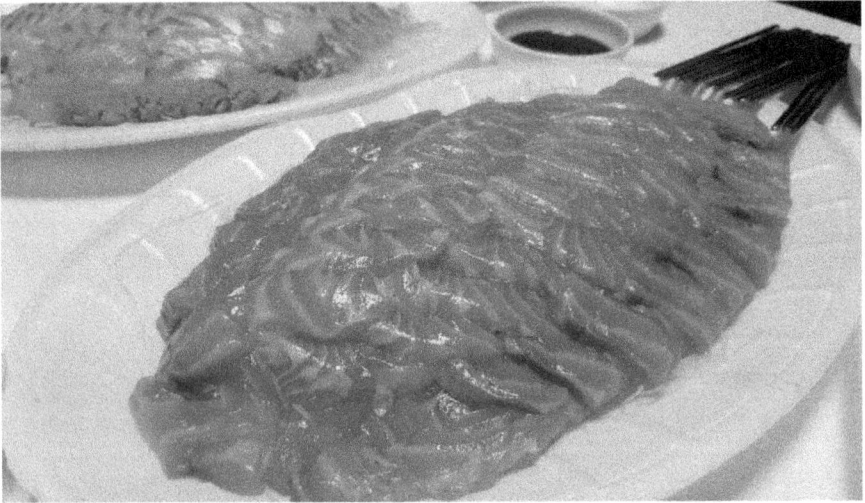

Tuna in crust

Ingredients:

600 grams of tuna steak sesame seeds pistachio oil breadcrumbs and salt

Description:

cut the slices of fresh tuna to the preferred size talk rest in a bowl brushed with oil aside, we combine the pistachios to sesame breadcrumbs and salt. For the moment then to take our slices of tuna pass them inside our crunchy beaten and seared 1 minute per side in a non-stick pan without oil.

Serve immediately, bon appetit.

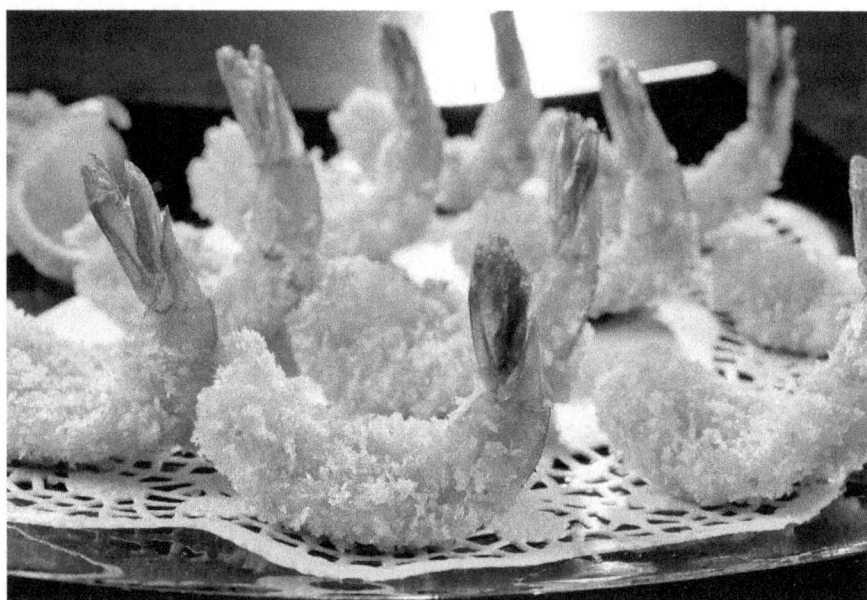

Shrimp Risotto

Ingredients:

- 350g of rice
- 400g of prawns
- ½ onion
- clove of garlic
- 2 glasses of white wine
- parsley
- 1 liter and 1/2 of broth
- salt and pepper

Description:

Clean the shrimps, fry the onion, garlic and shrimp heads, then add the white wine and cook for 10 minutes. Remove the shrimp heads and add the rice, after toasting it, add the fish stock like a normal risotto. After 8-9 minutes of cooking, add the cleaned shrimps and parsley and serve piping hot (do not add Parmesan cheese).

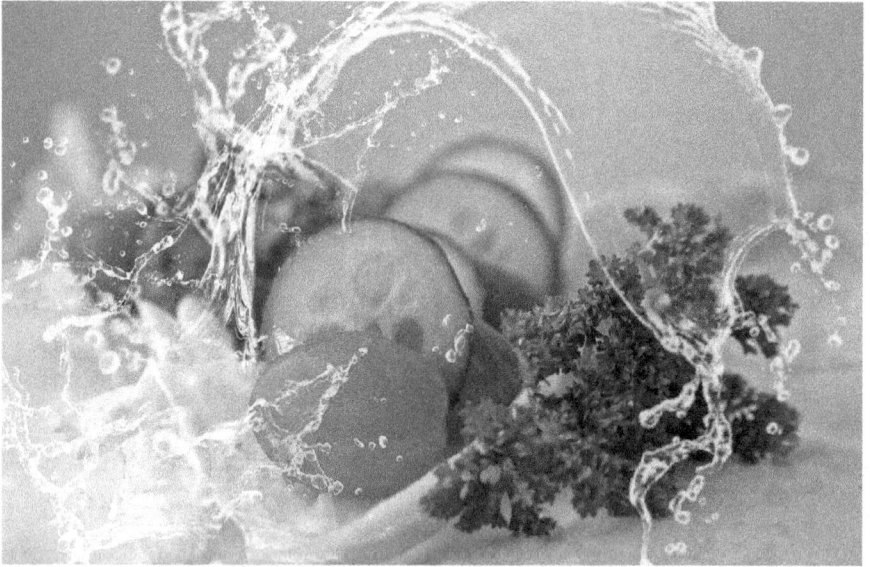

Rustic Macaroni

Ingredients:

- 350 g of macaroni
- 2 onions
- 2 fresh tomatoes
- parsley
- 1 ladle of broth
- 2 spoons of parmesan cheese
- salt and pepper

Description:

fry the onion, add the broth, then add the diced tomatoes, parsley and cheese and cook until the sauce is smooth cook the macaroni, drain and add to the sauce serve with grated Parmesan and freshly ground pepper

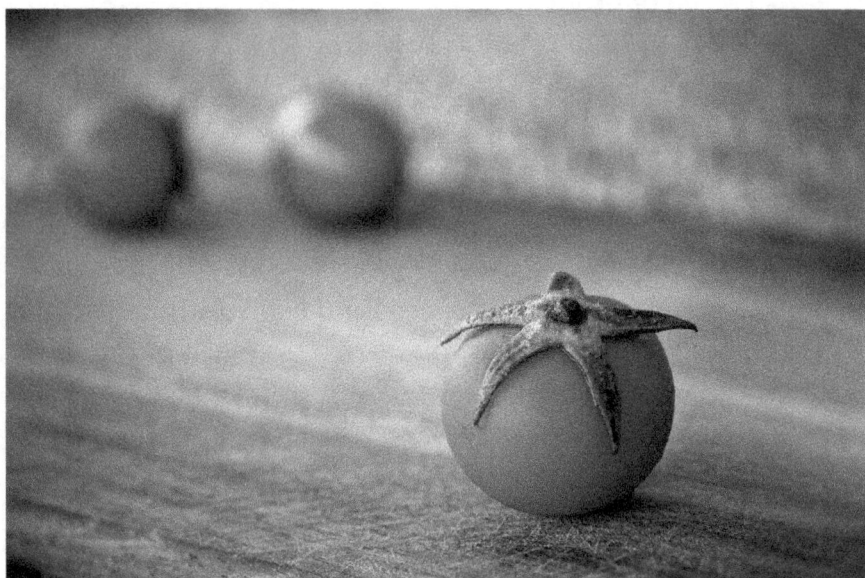

Spaghetti baked in foil

Ingredients:

- 350 g of spaghetti
- 300 g of tomatoes
- basil
- 1 garlic clove
- lemon juice
- capers
- salt and pepper

Description:

cook the spaghetti being careful to drain them al dente, keep 2-3 ladles of cooking water aside. after that, make small incisions in the skin of the tomatoes, immerse them in boiling water for a few minutes, and peel them, cut them and soak them in lemon juice, add the capers and cook over low heat for about twenty minutes. Add the finely chopped garlic and
basil and remove from the heat. Put the spaghetti with the sauce in a bowl and mix, apart from the spaghetti, prepare a sheet of paper with the sauce.

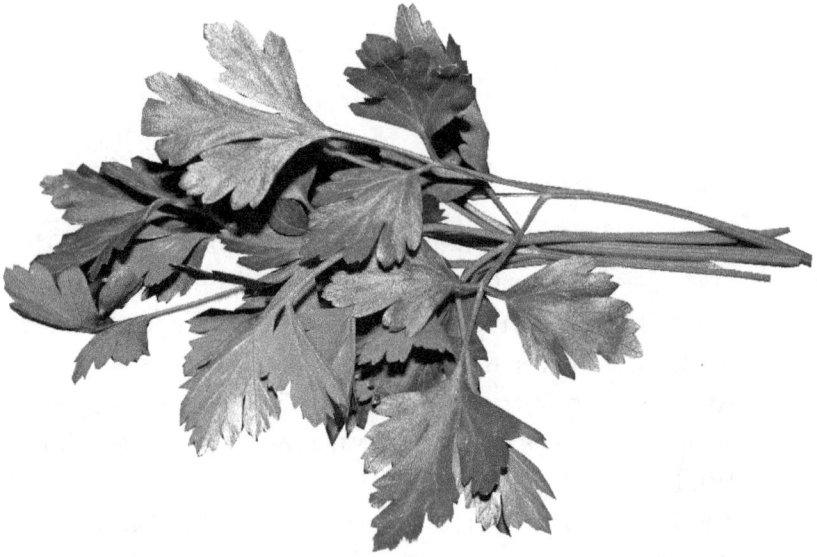

Rigatoni with Eggplant Sauce

Ingredients:

350 g rigatoni 1 eggplant 200 g peeled tomatoes 1/2 onion 1 clove of garlic 1 sprig of parsley 1 sprig of basil 200 g ricotta cheese Salt

Description:

dice the eggplant and leave it on a dish towel to dry completely, in a pot, create a fund of garlic onion 2 tablespoons of oil, when the onion begins to brown, lower the heat and add the eggplant and cook for 30 minutes. When cooked, add the parsley and basil to the sauce, well washed, with the stems removed and finely chopped. Cook the rigatoni in abundant salted water, drain well and set aside two pieces of pasta.

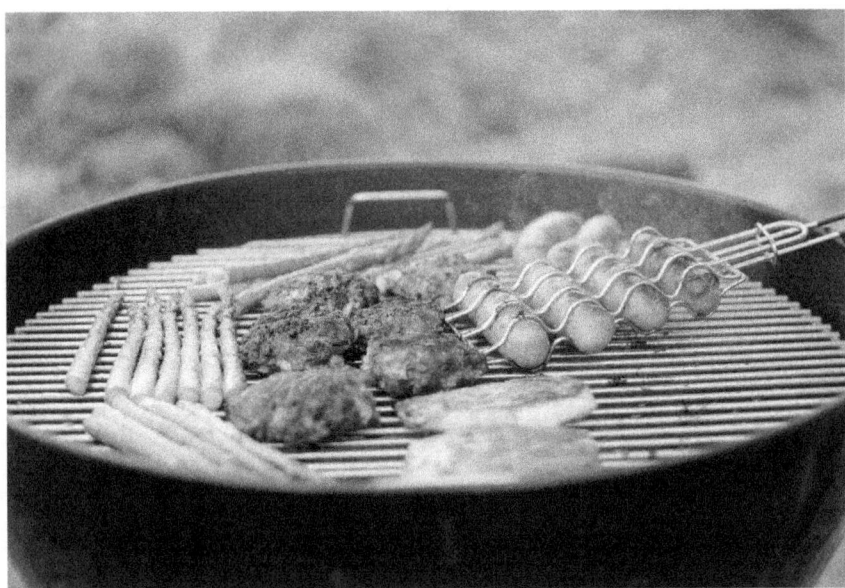

Low Fat Risotto with Curry

Ingredients:

1 kg of crustaceans Chopped garlic onion and parsley
1/2 glass of white wine Tomato sauce

Description:

polar of a gros boss 3 migon reagan, jomon - pada do make flavor lake, the onion clase teli cook for few minutes stirring well. Wet them with the site and when 2 sto will be evaporated, unite zest of the throats and the sauce of tomato cita in little water or the tomatoes peeled. Cover and cook a moment longer, then add the clams and shrimp and remove from heat after a few minutes. Separately cook the rice by
adding the broth poco at a time and at 3/4 of cooking time pour in all the prepared sauce and curry and sprinkle with Parmesan cheese. Curry is a mixture of spices, wisely dosed and carefully pounded, which includes cloves, nutmeg, mace, comino seeds, pepper, cardamom, cinnamon and saffron.

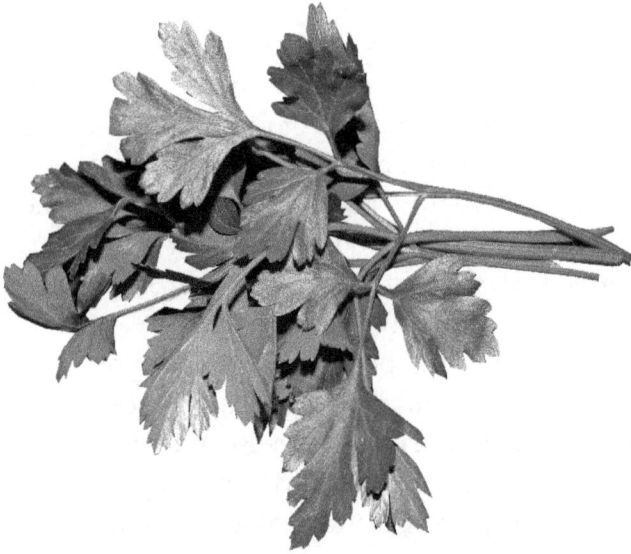

Lemon Sole

Ingredients:

400g sole fillets 2 lemons prosciutto ham anchovies 2 dl milk salt and pepper

Description:

Remove the peel from the lemons, taking care to also eliminate the white part, slice them and remove any seeds. Place the lemon slices on the bottom of an oven dish, then the anchovy fillets broken into pieces, the slices of prosciutto and lastly the sole fillets. Season everything with salt and pepper and bake in a hot oven at 240 °C for about 10 minutes. After this time, moisten everything with milk and keep in the oven for another 25 minutes. Remove from the oven, arrange the sole fillets on a serving plate, whisk the cooking juices and pour the resulting sauce over the fish. Serve piping hot.

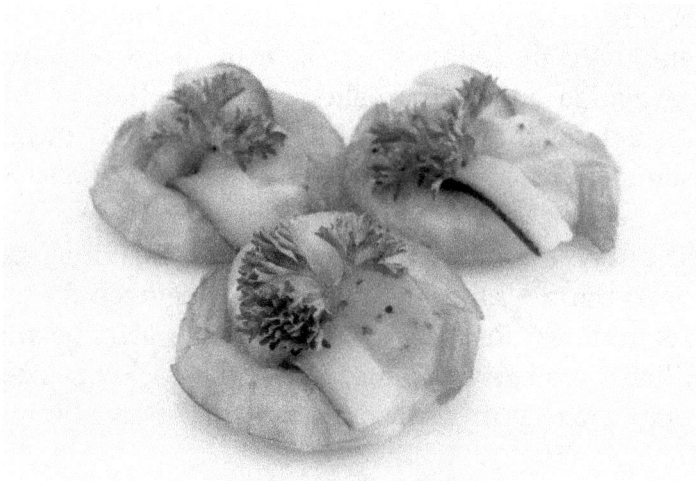

Roast Veal My Way

Ingredients:

- 15 gr of pine nuts
- 4 pitted green olives
- 60 gr of butter or margarine
- 600 gr of veal meat
- of black olives
- a ladle of broth
- salt and pepper

Description:

Take 10 g of butter or margarine and brown the pine nuts, then pound them in a mortar or with a meat pounder together with 4 pitted green olives. In 50 g of butter brown the veal meat, add the pine nuts and the crushed olives, the whole olives and the ladle of water. If the sauce is too much, remove the meat and let it reduce over high heat. Serve the meat in slices covered with the sauce and with the whole olives. Accompany the roast with spinach in butter or other vegetables to taste.

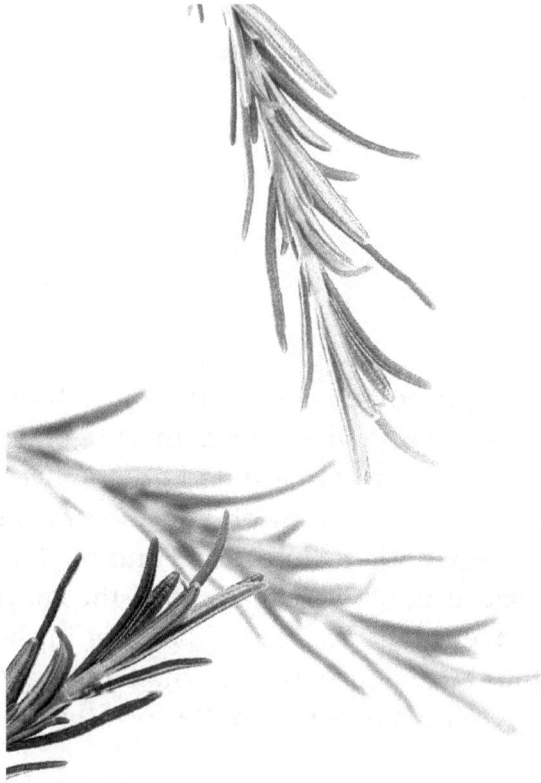

Escalope Valdostana style

Ingredients:

- 400 gr of sliced veal
- 150 gr of fontina cheese
- milk
- Bread in a box
- 60 gr of margarine

Description:

Beat the slices of meat well, remove the skins, score the edges and roll them in flour. In browned margarine, brown them on both sides, season with salt and pepper. On top of each slice place one of the fontina cheese, then sprinkle with milk, cover the pan and keep warm. Brown the slices of bread in the remaining margarine, arrange them on the serving plate, place the slices of meat on top and pour the cooking sauce over them. Serve immediately

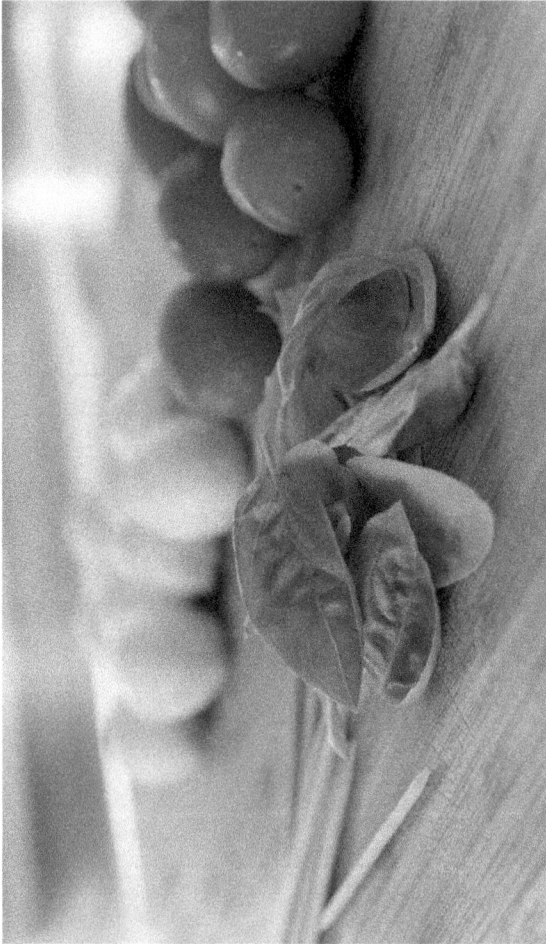

Veal in Jelly

Ingredients:

400 gr of sliced veal 80 gr of pork loin 80 gr of raw ham half a clove of garlic 50 gr of breadcrumbs milk 1 egg yolk lemon zest sage grated parmesan nutmeg 80 gr of butter flour stock cube 1 liter of jelly salt and pepper

Description:

On the beaten meat slices, about 12x6 cm wide, spread with the blade of a knife the following stuffing: pass twice in the mincer the pork loin, the ham, the garlic and the breadcrumbs soaked in milk and squeezed; mix the egg yolk and the lemon rind, the Parmesan cheese, salt, pepper, nutmeg and mix everything well. Roll up the slices of meat thus prepared, joined two by two with a sage leaf in between and stick them on two toothpicks. Take care that the mexicans are well closed. Melt the butter in a pan, add the lightly floured Mexicans and let them brown on all sides. Pour in a little broth, cover and cook slowly for about 3/4 hour until the sauce is well reduced. Remove them, place them on absorbent paper and let them cool completely. Place them in a deep dish and cover them with the warm but liquid jelly. Keep the dish in the refrigerator for a few hours before serving.

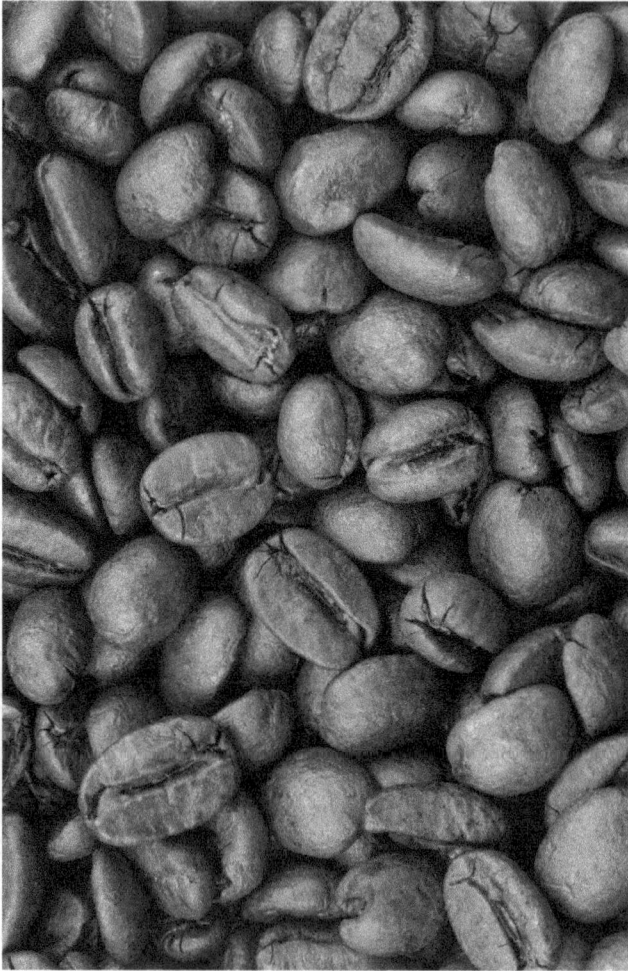

Veal and Green Beans Salad

Ingredients:

300 gr green beans 1 bell pepper 500 gr veal carrot celery stalk 1/2 onion salt

Description:

Put the piece of meat in a saucepan with the carrot, celery, onion, a little salt and water; let everything cook for about 2 hours, then drain the piece of meat and in the broth cook the green beans for about 25 minutes from the beginning of boiling. Drain these too with a slotted spoon and place them in a bowl with the diced meat. On the flame directly toast the bell pepper, remove the burnt skin and cut it into strips. Add it to the other ingredients, stir well and season with the green sauce softened and worked together with 2 tablespoons of meat cooking broth.

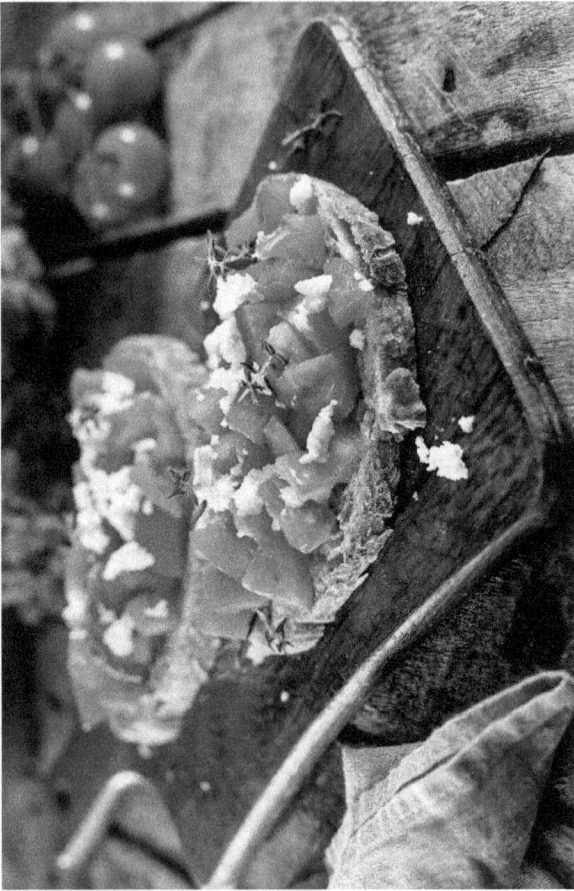

Involtini Trevisani

Ingredients:

300g rump of veal trevisana 50g margarine 4 slices of cheese 1/2 glass of white wine flour sage salt and pepper

Description:

Wash the trevisana, cut it into four vertically and brown the tufts obtained in a pan with 25 g of margarine and a pinch of salt. On top of each slice of veal place a slice of cheese and a tuft of trevisana. In a frying pan, melt the remaining margarine, add the sage leaves and the roulades, leave to gain flavor for a few moments, season with salt and pepper and sprinkle with white wine. Cover and cook over low heat for about 20 minutes, diluting if necessary with a little stock.

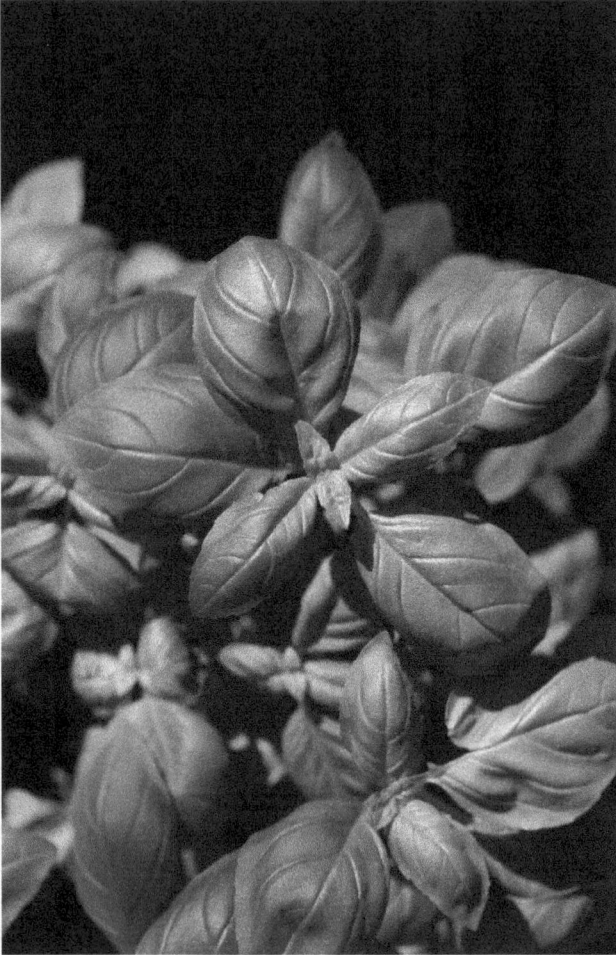

Stuffed Escalope

Ingredients:

600 g veal 60 g ham 200 g minced pork aromatic herbs shallot cognac 4 eggs Butter salt and pepper.

Description:

Have your trusted butcher prepare a nice slice of veal, beating it well to half an inch thick. Prepare with the aromatic herbs, eggs, pepper, a nice omelette and spread it on the escalope. Cover it with the slices of ham. Mix the pork with the shallot or minced garlic, cognac, salt and pepper and place it in the center of the escalope, giving the shape of a small salami. Roll the whole on itself, sew with a large white thread and proceed to roast in the pot seasoning with a little salt and pepper and sprinkling with a little broth if necessary, or with a little hot water. Cook everything for about an hour with the lid on and serve the escalope in slices.

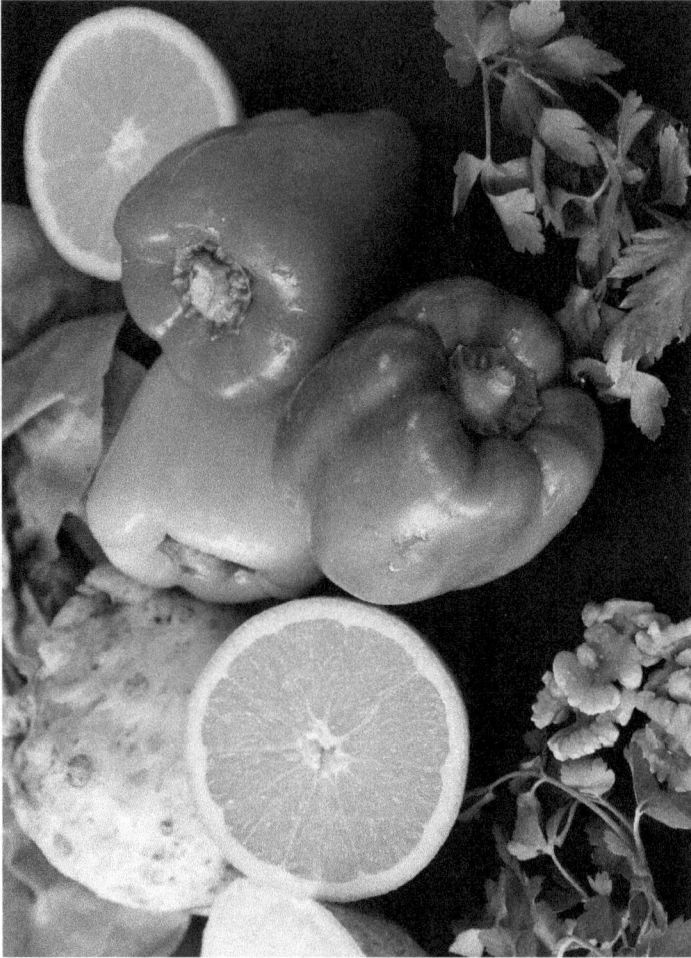

Spicy Veal

Ingredients:

400 g veal meat 50 g butter 100 g artichokes mushrooms and gherkins ½ glass white wine 1 liter broth salt and pepper

Description:

In a pan, brown the butter, add the slices of meat and cook for 15 minutes on each side without browning them, then remove them and arrange them on a plate. In the sauce left in the pan put the white wine, artichokes, mushrooms and gherkins coarsely chopped together. Let it cook for 2 or 3 minutes then put the meat back in. Season with salt and pepper and add a glass of stock, cover and continue cooking slowly for 20 minutes. Add broth from time to time if necessary and serve the slices with their reduced sauce.

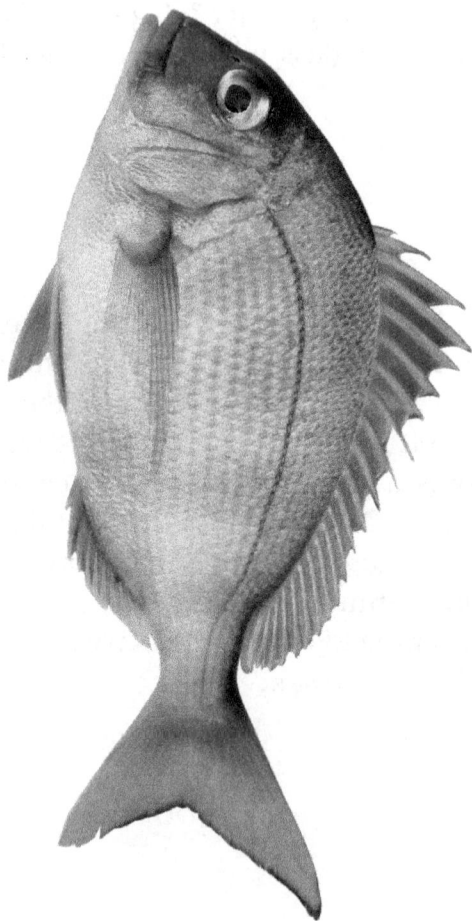

Veal Stew

Ingredients:

50 gr butter Chopped onion 600 gr veal stew White wine 250 gr peeled tomatoes 400 gr shelled peas Flour Salt and pepper Nutmeg stock

Description:

Brown the spring onion in butter, add the lightly floured stews and let them brown, then season with salt, pepper and nutmeg. Sprinkle with dry white wine and, when it has evaporated, add the peeled tomatoes and a few ladles of broth. Cover and leave for about half an hour, then add the peas and finish cooking, pouring more broth if necessary. If you are using preserved peas, add them just before the end of cooking.

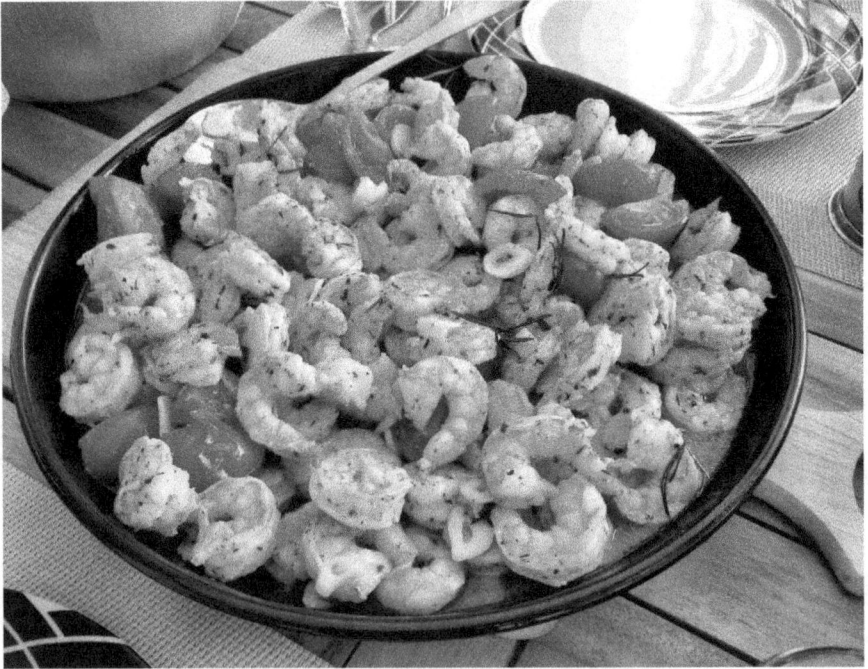

Cotolette alla Palermitana

Ingredients:

400 gr of veal rump 2 eggs breadcrumbs 5 slices of cheese parsley 30 gr of flour 1/2 liter of milk 1/2 glass of marsala 130 gr of margarine salt

Description:

With the flour, 30 g of margarine, a pinch of salt and the milk, prepare a béchamel sauce that is not too thick. Then add an egg yolk and chopped parsley, as soon as it has cooled a little. Dip the veal slices first in the egg and then in the breadcrumbs and cook them like normal cutlets in the remaining margarine. Place the cutlets in an oven-proof dish, season with a pinch of salt, sprinkle with Marsala wine, lay the slices of cheese on top and cover with the béchamel sauce. Bake in the oven for about 20 minutes and then serve.

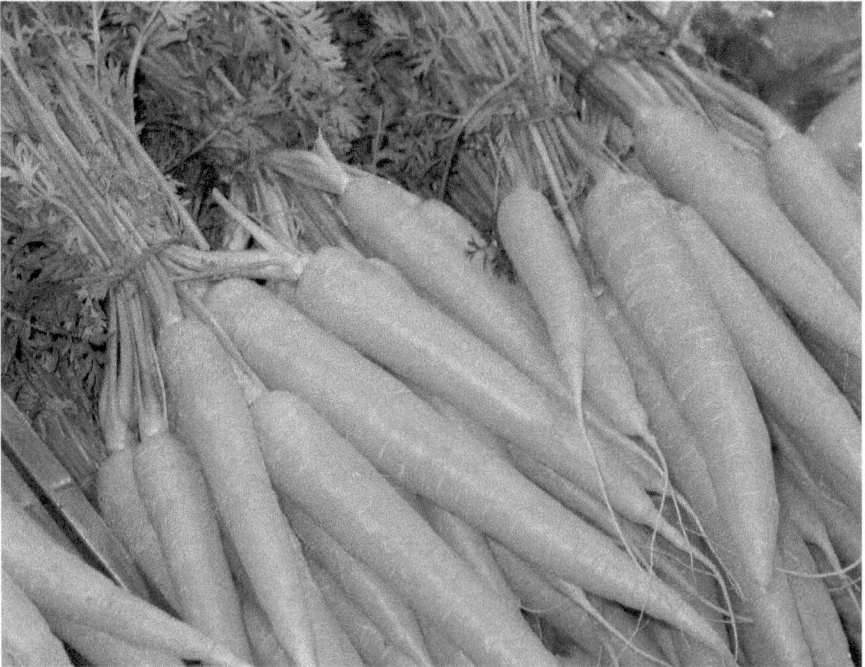

Italian style sea bream

Ingredients:

1 rata weighing 1 kg 100 g of cultivated mushrooms 60 g of butter a glass of vermouth two tablespoons of liquid cream 30 g of Parmesan cheese 20 g of breadcrumbs 20 g of flour half an onion 1 clove of garlic a bay leaf parsley salt and pepper

Description:

remove the head and tail from the gilthead and divide it into 4, put the head and tail together with the onion, garlic and bay leaf, salt and a glass of water and cook for 30 minutes in a pot over medium heat. Filter the mixture and set it aside, turn on the heat under a frying pan and put the fish stock that you have already filtered and place the 4 slices of gilthead on top, add the vermouth and a glass of water seasoned with salt and leave for 20 minutes over low heat. Drain the fish, remove the skin, remove the bones and place in an oven-proof dish. Melt 30 g of butter, add the flour and half a ladle of cooking stock and bring to the boil, stirring occasionally, then add the sauce with the chopped mushrooms, chopped parsley and a little salt and pepper, a little at a time, then add the fish stock and place in the oven, sprinkling a layer of breadcrumbs on top.

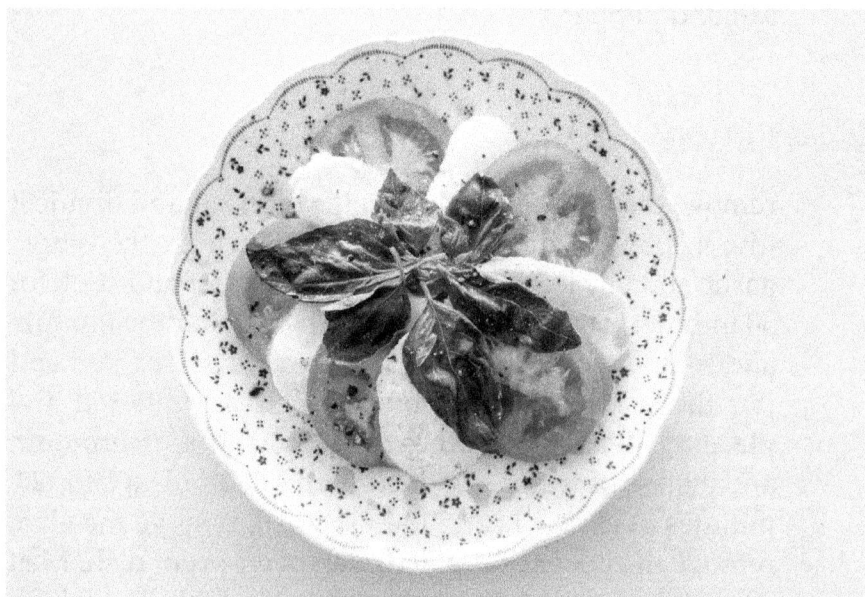

Baked sea bream

Ingredients:

1 kilo and two pound gilthead half a glass of oil two cloves of garlic half an onion 300 grams of tomatoes a glass and a half of white wine marjoram and thyme parsley salt and pepper

Description:

Clean prepare the sea bream to be cooked then eviscerate it remove the scales clean the gills and create transverse incisions on the entire belly is prepared on one side and the other then a pyrex dish suitable for the oven make a fund of oil garlic chopped onion Add the washed tomatoes, skinned and cut into pieces, add the marjoram, thyme, salt and pepper to taste and place them on top of the sea bream. Add the parsley, washed and finely chopped, a glass of wine and leave in a hot oven for 30 minutes, turning occasionally.

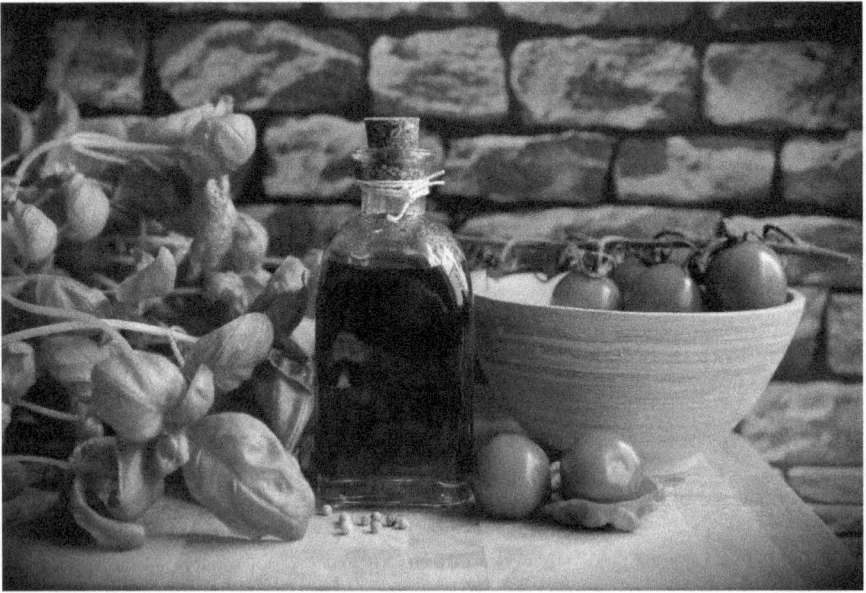

Branzino Branzino in white wine

Ingredients:

a 1 kg sea bass 50 grams of butter 30 grams of breadcrumbs a hard-boiled egg a fresh onion a glass of white wine a bay leaf parsley a head of garlic salt pepper and half a liter of fish stock

Description:

Carefully clean the sea bass, remove the scales, remove the entrails, remove the fins and wash it well under cold running water. Remove the hips The central bone and then obtain two equal fillets seasoned with salt and pepper aside mix the breadcrumbs with the fresh onion already chopped the butter the yolk of an egg
chopped parsley and mix well with this filled the sea bass then place the sea bass in an ovenproof dish add the white wine and mix well. the sea bass in an ovenproof dish wet it with white wine add the broth that you have obtained by boiling half a
liter of water with the entrails and bones of the sea bass itself sprinkle the sea bass in the dish with the bus with its broth is left for 40 minutes in the oven

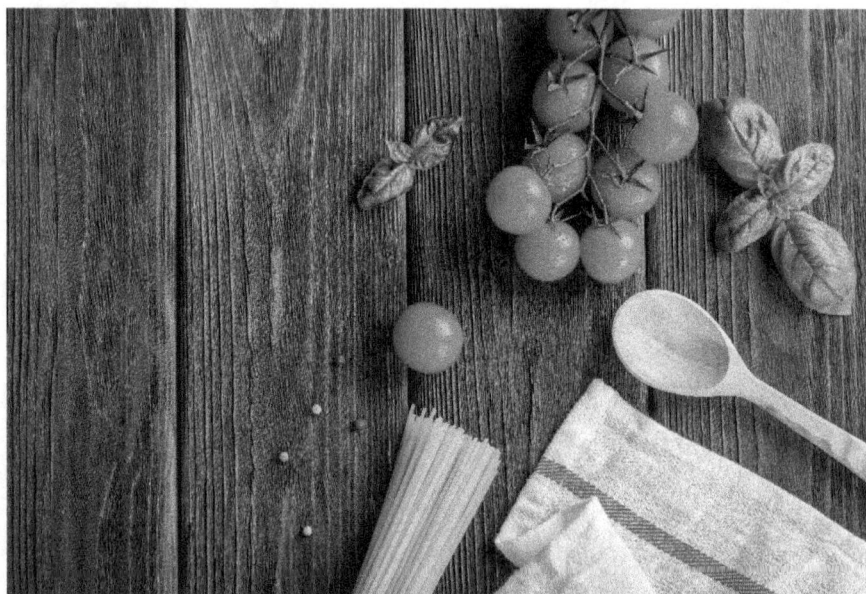

Sea bass baked in foil

Ingredients:

one and a half kilo of sea bass one lemon 2 tablespoons of oil 200 g of mushrooms rosemary garlic salt and pepper

Description:

Wash and eviscerate the sea bass under running water and let it dry. Soak the dried mushrooms in water for about 40 minutes, then drain them and cut them finely. Take some greaseproof paper and put it on top of the sea bass, season with lemon juice, oil and parsley. At this point, close the greaseproof paper on itself, creating a cartoccio, place the fish with all its liquid in an oven-proof dish and cook for 35 minutes at 220°.

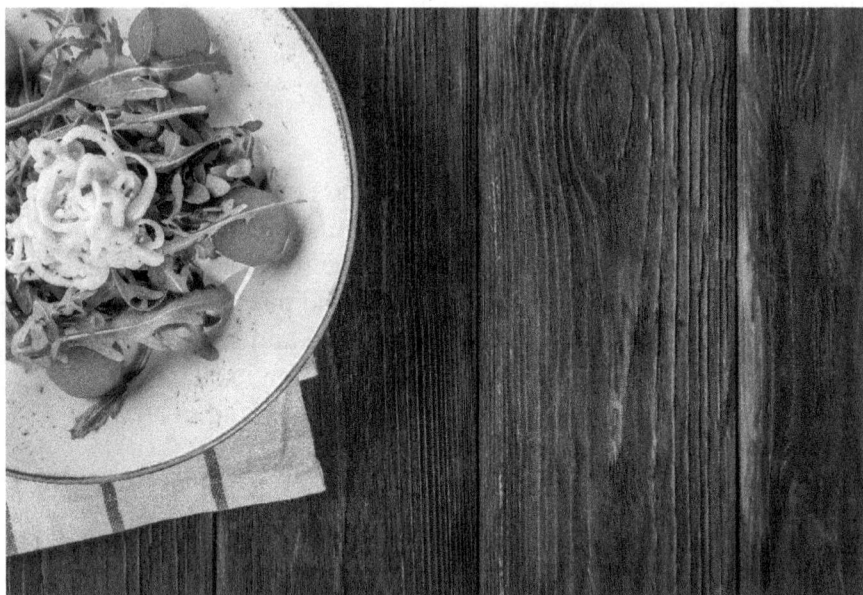

Sea bass in salt

Ingredients:

one sea bass weighing one kilo and two kilograms coarse salt about one and a half kilograms two or three lemons rosemary leaves and parsley

Description:

Clean the sea bass, remove the entrails, leave the head and the tail, put them in a pan with high sides, about 1 cm of coarse salt, put the sea bass on top, add the parsley and the rosemary and cover it with the lemon slices and then add the rest of the coarse salt until the sea bass is completely covered, then put it in the oven at 250 degrees for 30 minutes, serve with parsley and lemon juice if desired.

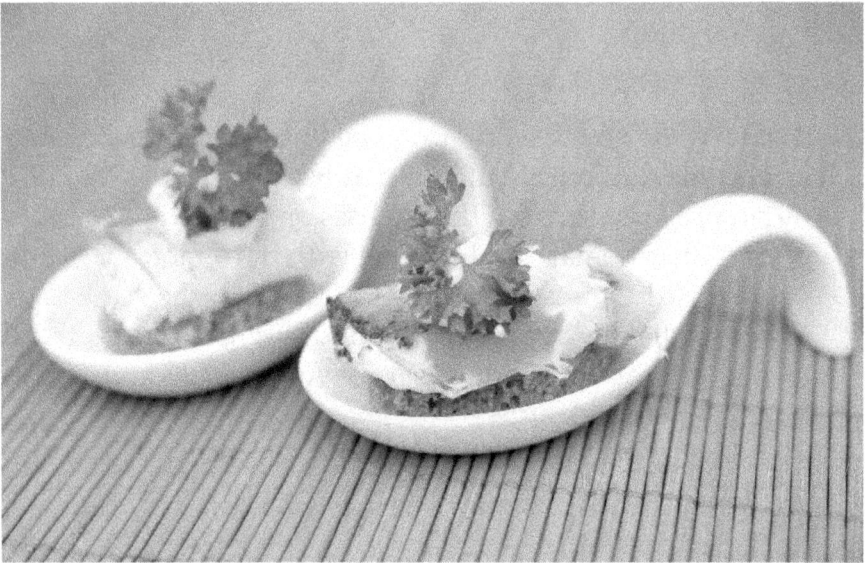

Spinach Puree

Ingredients:

600 g potatoes; 400 g spinach I bunch of watercress 60 g butter; 4 tablespoons grated Parmesan cheese 1/2 1 of milk 2 egg whites 2 tablespoons whipped cream I knob of butter salt

Description:

Boil the potatoes in their skins, wash the spinach thoroughly and put it in a pot and add a handful of coarse salt; let it cook for 10 minutes over medium heat. Put the spinach in the blender and add the watercress leaves, obtaining a thick mush. After peeling the potatoes, mash them in a potato masher. Over low heat, mash the spinach mixture to evaporate all the water
and then add the butter cut into small pieces. Using an electric whisk, mix in the spinach puree a little at a time and add the hot milk a little at a time. Let the puree dry and swell and it will take on a nice light green color; add the grated Parmesan cheese and, if necessary. Whip the egg whites to stiff peaks and add them to the mixture; whip the cream, without sugaring it, and incorporate it. Bake in the oven for 15-20 minutes at 180 degrees.

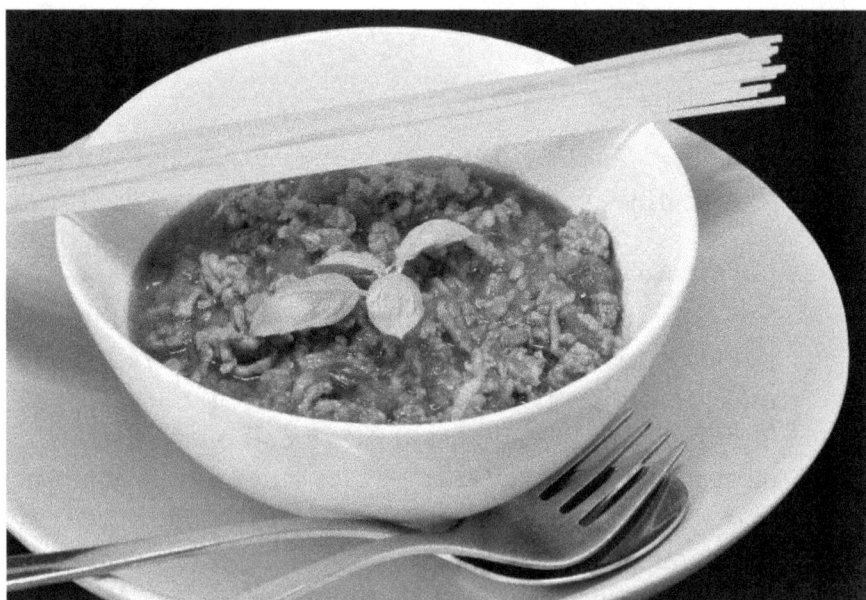

Liver in wine

Ingredients:

- 600 g of veal liver cut into slices
- 2 large onions
- 100 g of peeled tomatoes
- ½ glass of white wine
- 1 stock cube
- a little flour
- salt and pepper.

Description:

Sauté onions cut into half moons and dice (3-4 minutes)
add the tomatoes, season with salt and pepper and cook
over medium heat for 20 minutes flour the liver and cook
it together with the tomatoes
add ½ glass of white wine and let it evaporate serve the
liver covered with onions and tomatoes

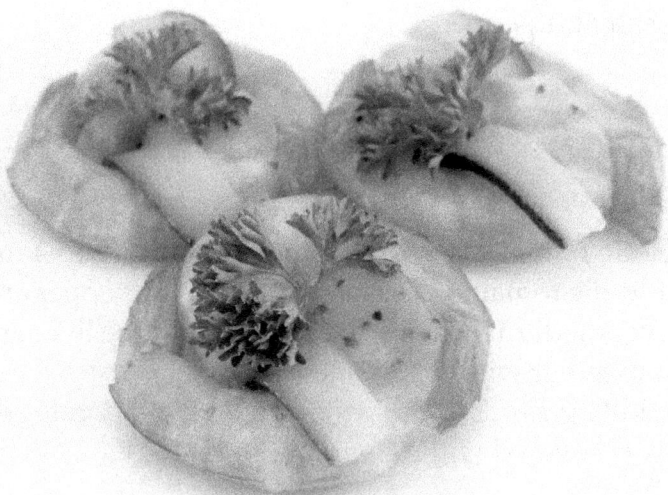

Meatballs

Ingredients:

400 g of minced beef 100 g of breadcrumbs soaked in milk and squeezed 2 eggs 2 tablespoons of grated Parmesan cheese 1 tablespoon of chopped parsley 200 g of peeled tomatoes 1 tablespoon of pine nuts 1 clove of garlic 2 teaspoons of sugar 2 tablespoons of vinegar 1/2 cube salt and pepper

Description:

In a bowl, add the meat, the breadcrumbs, the parsley, the eggs, the grated Parmesan cheese and a pinch of salt and pepper. Using your hands, create small balls and dip them first in the beaten egg yolk and then in the breadcrumbs. Heat a non-stick pan and add the peeled tomatoes. After 20 minutes over medium heat, add the meatballs, pine nuts to taste, salt and pepper to taste, cover and cook for about
25 minutes. Remove the lid and turn up the heat to evaporate the liquid.

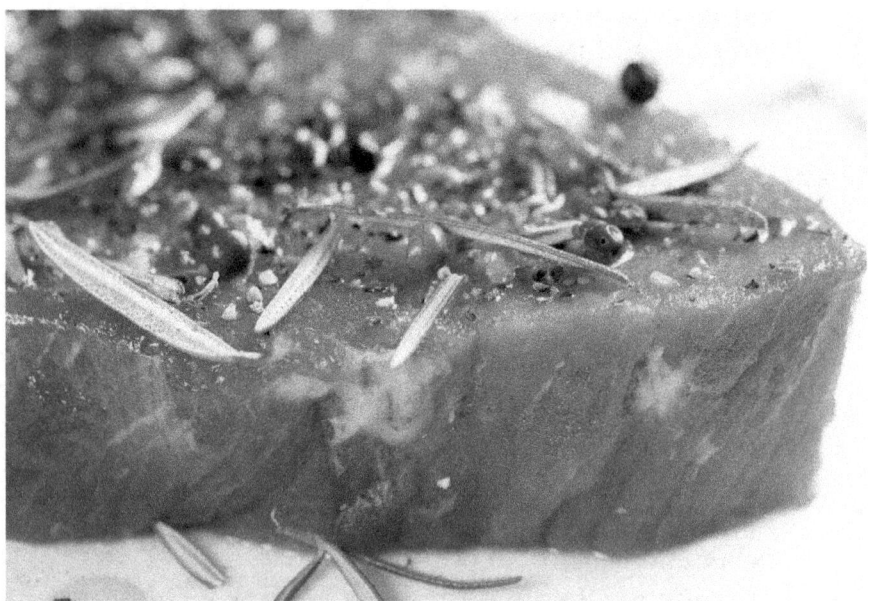

Bread basket with mushrooms

Ingredients:

1 round loaf of bread, not too big 800 g mushrooms 40 g dried mushrooms 2 eggs 1 sprig of parsley 1 clove of garlic 1 ladle of broth 1 dl milk 30 g grated Parmesan cheese salt and pepper the juice of 1/2 lemon

cut ¼ of the way up the bread (starting from the top) and hollow out the breadcrumbs.

Description:

in a bowl, place the dried mushrooms and let them soak for at least 20 minutes wash and slice the mushrooms lengthwise. Chop the garlic and dried mushrooms and brown them in a pot with a couple of ladles of broth. Add the lemon juice to the mushrooms and season with salt and pepper.
Let cook on low heat for 30 minutes with lid. Whisk together eggs and grana cheese, milk and chopped parsley.
Create a glossy and smooth mixture. Add the mushrooms and put the mixture in the basket of bread put in oven at 200 degrees for 20 minutes.

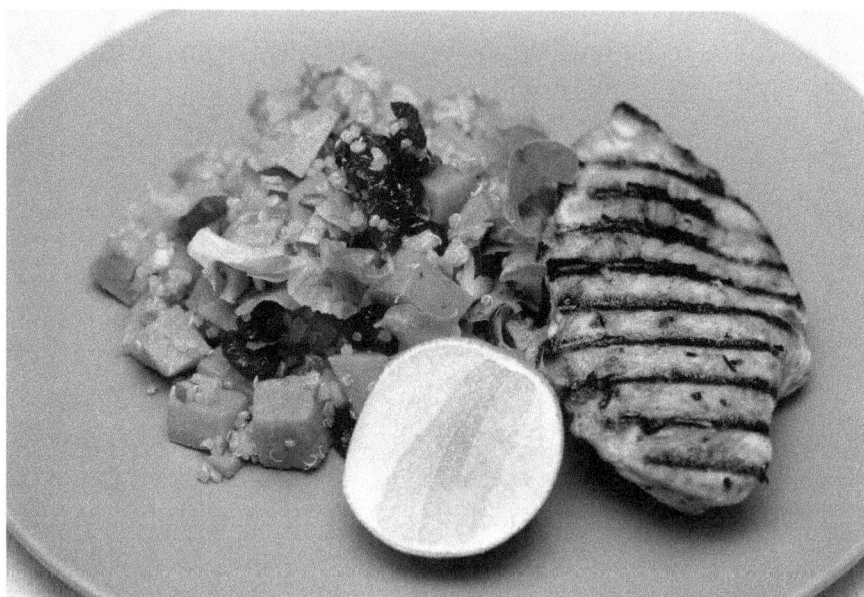

Veal and eggplant pie

Ingredients:

3 eggplants 1/2 onion 1 celery stalk 1 carrot 300 g minced veal 1 ladle of broth 200 g peeled tomatoes 200 g mozzarella 1 baslico cape 1/2 biochamber of wine grated parmesan salt, pepper

Description:

Wash and slice eggplant 1cm thick creating eggplant rounds; let drain on a dish towel for at least 15 minutes. Grill the eggplant using a very hot rimmed grill pan. (no oil or butter)
Chop onion celery and carrots sauté over medium heat for 3-4 minutes. Brown the meat and peeled tomatoes in it. Leave to cook over a low heat for 1 hour.
Line a mold with the grilled eggplant slices. Fill with the meat adding the mozzarella and some spices. Put a layer of grana cheese. 10-15 minutes in a ventilated oven at 200 degrees.
serve steaming

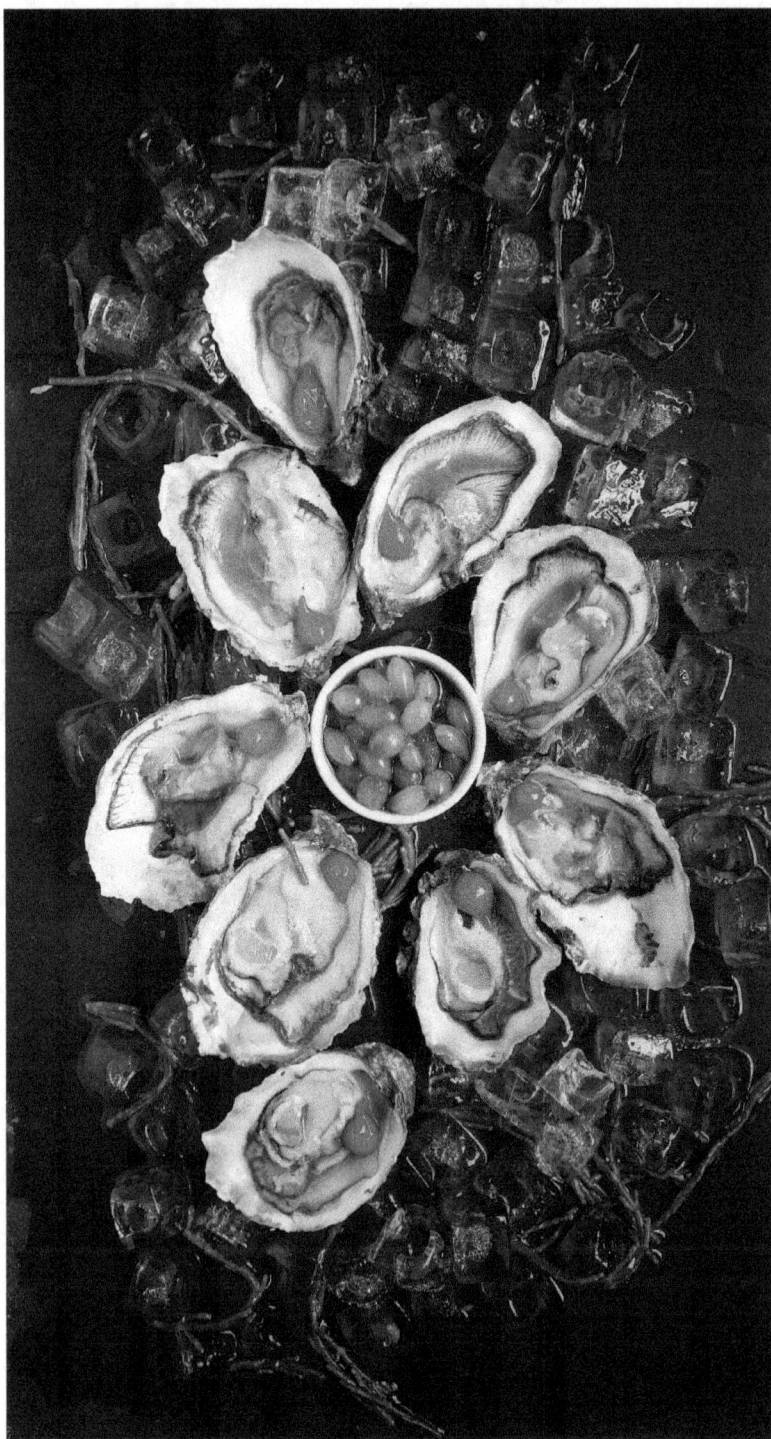

Veal with Parsley

Ingredients:

800 g veal rump in one piece 1 sprig of parsley the juice of 2 lemons 1 teaspoon of flour 2 ladles of stock the zest of 1/2 lemon grated a few leaves of sage 1 clove of garlic salt; freshly ground pepper

Description:

mince garlic, sage, add salt and pepper and place the meat slices on both sides (the mince should stick to the meat slices)

brown the meat slices on a medium heat, when it starts to brown add the lemon juice and a ladle of broth and let it cook on a low heat for 20 minutes

place the meat on a cutting board and cut it into slices arrange them on the serving plate adding the parsley and the zest of a lemon

Make a slurry with the remaining stock, when it is reduced enough pour it over the meat and serve.

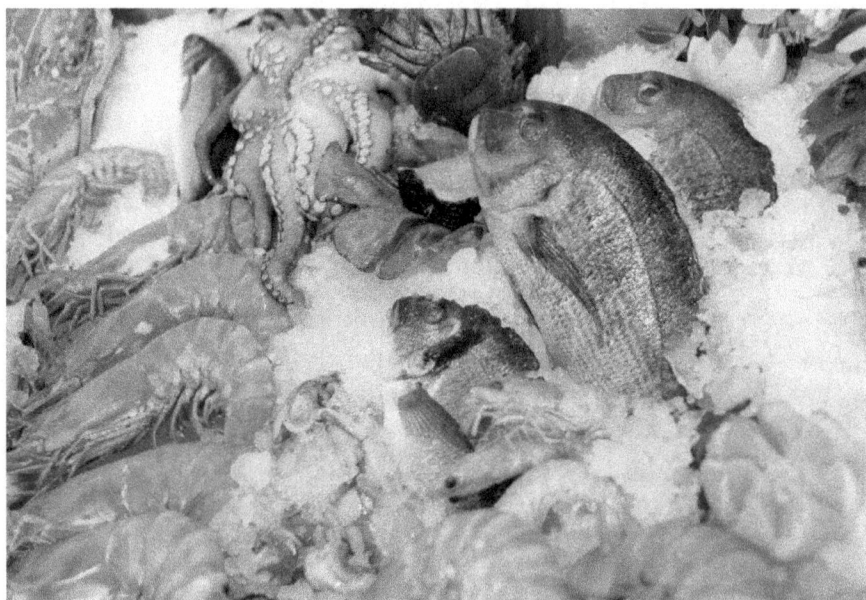

Hamburger with sauce

Ingredients:

4 hamburgers thick enough 1 carrot 2 onions 1 celery stalk 1/2 glass of red wine 400 g peeled tomatoes 1 pinch of sweet paprika 1 ladle of broth Salt Flour to taste

Description:

chop celery, onions and carrots, sauté for a few minutes then add a ladleful of broth. Let the broth evaporate and add the peeled tomatoes. Cook over medium heat for 25 minutes. Create the burgers and dip them in white 00 flour then place them in a hot pan, season with salt and pepper, turn them over and let them cook for 3 minutes on each side, then add the tomatoes, lower the heat and leave them for 15 minutes and serve.

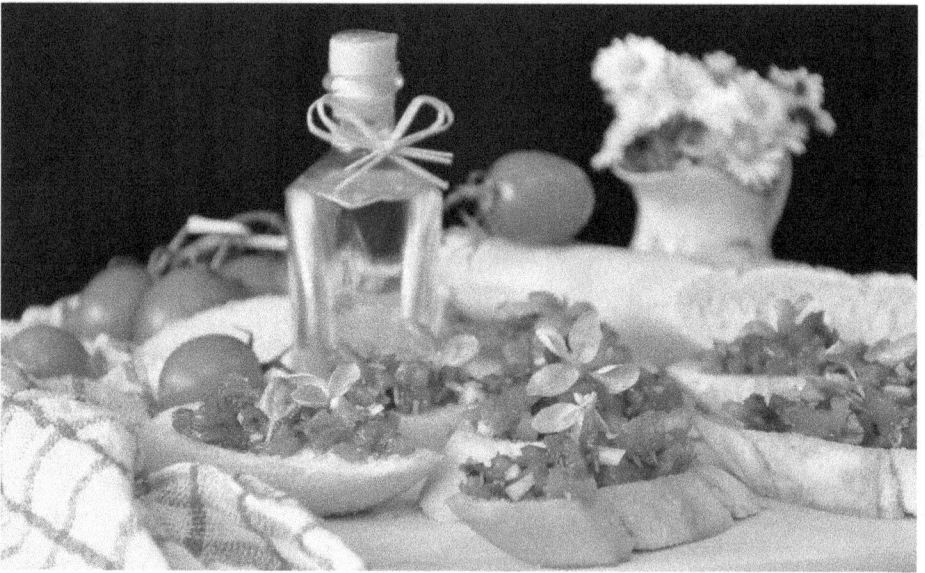

Stuffed zucchinis in guazzetto

Ingredients:

4 zucchinis, rather large and regular in shape 100 g cooked ham 1 egg 2 tablespoons grated Parmesan cheese 1/2 onion 1 tuft of parsley Breadcrumbs as needed 400 g peeled tomatoes salt and pepper

Description:

Clean the zucchini, wash them, remove the tops and bottoms and cut them in half to obtain 8 equal length pieces. Boil them in a little salted water; drain and empty them using a small digger. Put the zucchini pulp in a bowl with the egg, the grated Parmesan cheese, a little salt and pepper, the chopped cooked ham and enough breadcrumbs to mix everything together.

Stuff the zucchini with the mixture. In a casserole put the onion and parsley finely chopped, add the chopped tomatoes and put everything on the fire. Adjust salt and pepper and after 15 minutes put the zucchini in the casserole. Let them cook for another 10 minutes and serve hot or warm according to your taste.

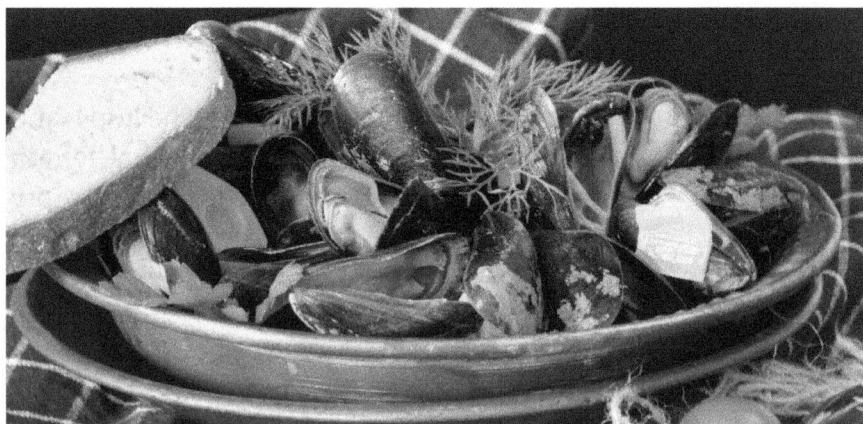

Canapes with peas

Ingredients:

8 milk sandwiches 1 egg 40 g Emmental 100 g canned peas 1/2 onion 50 g cooked ham 3 tablespoons milk salt

Description:

Fry the finely chopped onion in a saucepan, as soon as it turns golden, add the milk with the peas and the cooked ham in pieces Season with a pinch of salt and cook over low heat for about 20 minutes. Whip the egg whites until stiff and add the Parmesan cheese to the yolk, then add the peas and the ham to the yolk. Once mixed well, add the egg whites without disassembling them and put them inside the milk buns and bake for 15 minutes at 200 degrees.

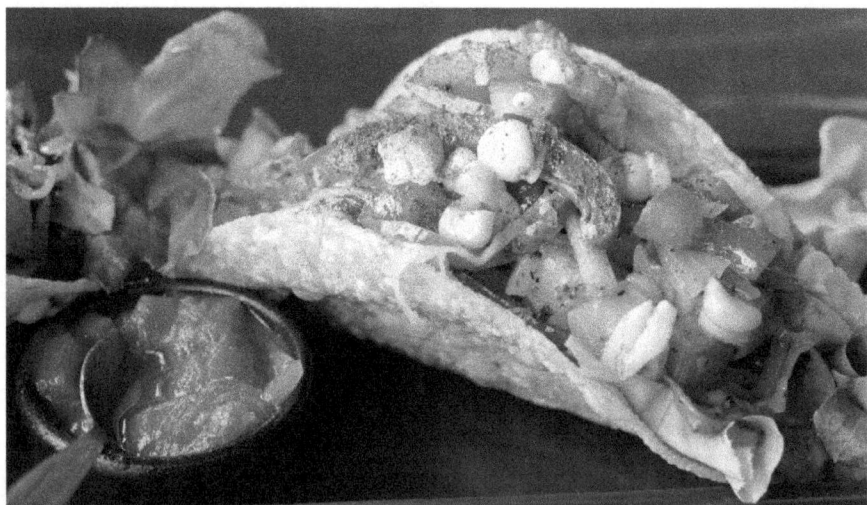

Lemon Sole

Ingredients:

4 soles 6 tablespoons meat stock 2 tablespoons vinegar juice of 1 lemon 2 tablespoons white wine 2 cloves 2 bay leaves 1 onion Salt pepper

Description:

remove the heads and tails from the sole, chop the garlic, onion, lemon juice, 1 ladle of broth, the vinegar and the wine, blend everything and set aside 1 cup of the mixture, place the remaining liquid in an ovenproof dish and add the fish, season with salt and pepper. After 10 minutes of cooking, add the remaining liquid. After another 10 minutes, turn on a frying pan and finish cooking the sole; the pan will give the fish a nice golden color.

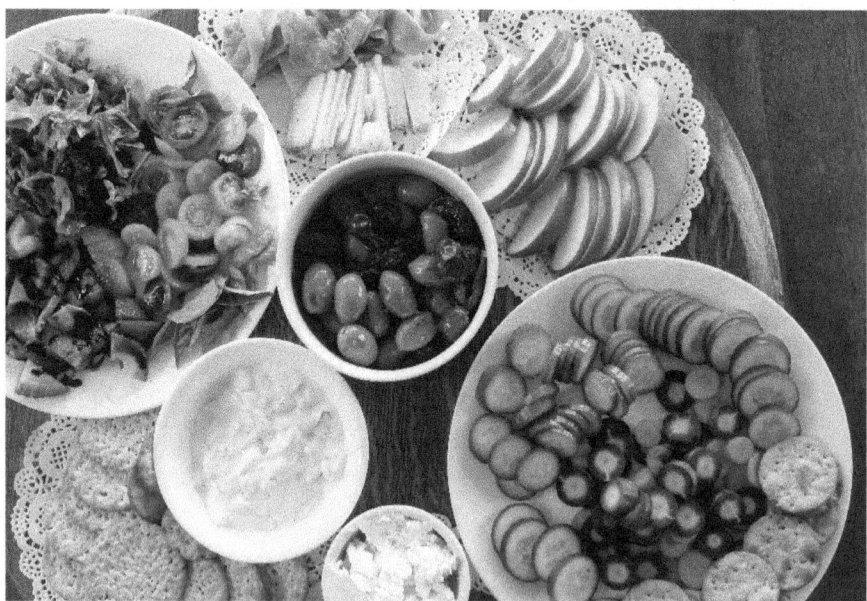

Ricotta and spinach pie

Ingredients:

- 400 g of frozen spinach
- 200 g of ricotta cheese
- 2 whole eggs
- 1 egg white
- 40g of parmesan cheese
- 1 pinch of nutmeg
- salt
- pepper

Description:

chop the spinach and add the ricotta cheese, season with grated nutmeg, salt and pepper, also add the yolks of eggs and parmesan cheese, make the mixture smooth and homogeneous aside mount the egg whites and incorporate them being careful not to disassemble put everything in an oven dish and cook at 200 degrees for 45 minutes when the torino will be nice and golden, serve hot

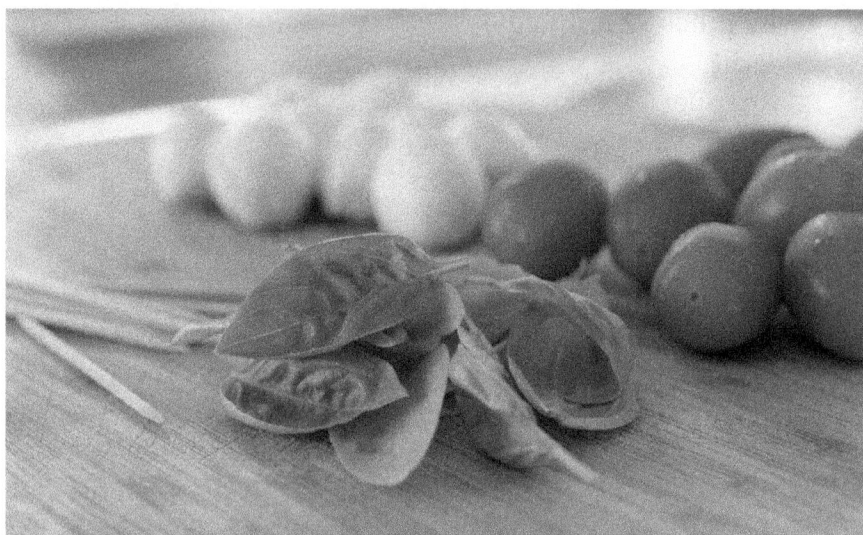

seafood polenta

Ingredients:

8 slices of polenta 300 g shrimps 300 g mussels 300 g
baby octopus 1/2 onion 1 clove of garlic 3 tablespoons
dry white wine 1 pinch of chili pepper 1 tuft of basil 2
tablespoons stock 3 ripe tomatoes 1 tuft of parsley salt

Description:

toast the polenta made in slices on a ribbed steak pan chop the
parsley garlic put them in a pot with 2 fingers of water, add the
mussels and shrimps, cover and turn on the fire. After a short
time the mussels will be open, shell the mussels and shrimps.
Sauté the onions and garlic, add the cleaned baby octopus, add
a glass of white wine, add the diced tomatoes and cook for 30
minutes over medium heat, then add the mussels and shrimp,
parsley, lemon and basil. Place the shellfish on the polenta and
drizzle with the broth.

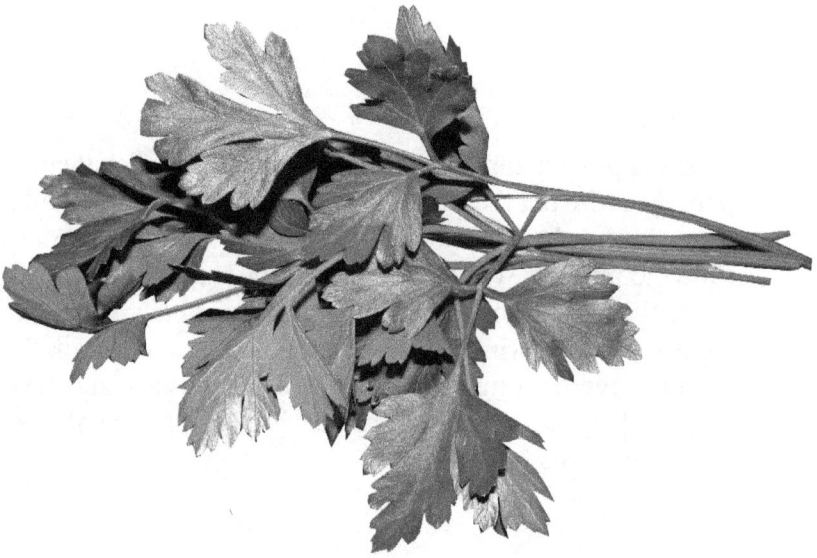

Crown of rice with peas

Ingredients:

350 g of rice 1 kg of fresh peas 1 onion 80 g of uncooked ham 1 tuft of parsley 1 liter and 1/2 of broth 3 tablespoons of grated Parmesan cheese Salt pepper

Description:

Sauté finely chopped onions, place them in two different pots, add a ladle of broth in both pots and cook. In one of the two pots, add the ham cut into pieces with the peas and cook for 40 minutes in the second pot, add the rice and cook it for 15 minutes, adding broth if necessary.

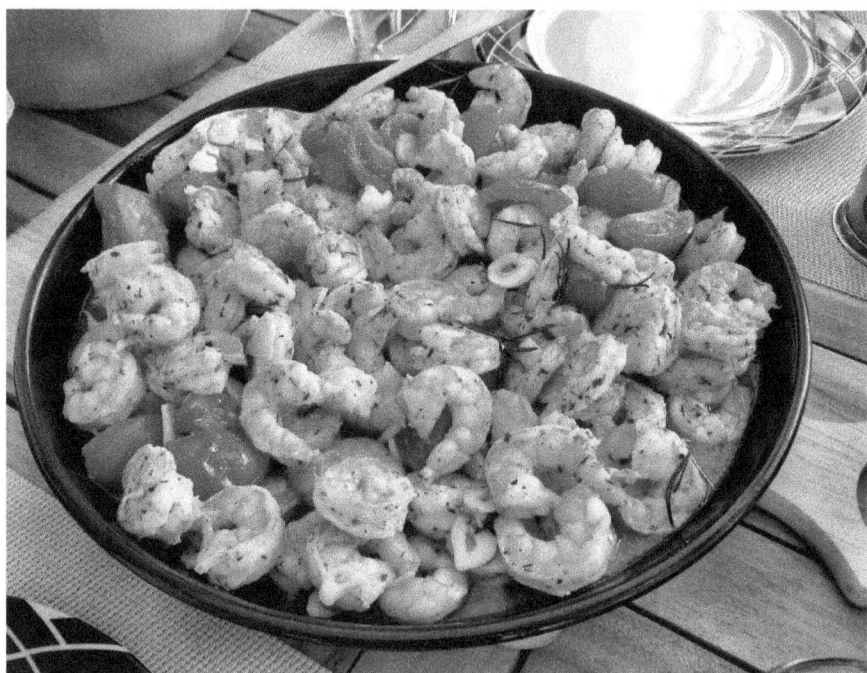

Braised peas

Ingredients:

1 kg of fresh peas
a few leaves of lettuce
100 g of baby onions
50 g of ham
2 ladles of broth
Pepper

Description:

Shell the peas, slice the spring onions and cut the lettuce and ham into strips. Put everything together in a non-stick saucepan and brown lightly over high heat, stirring constantly with a wooden spoon. Then add the broth, lower the heat, cover and let everything cook for about 30 minutes, stirring occasionally. When cooked, add the sauce, if necessary; add pepper to taste, remove from heat and serve immediately.

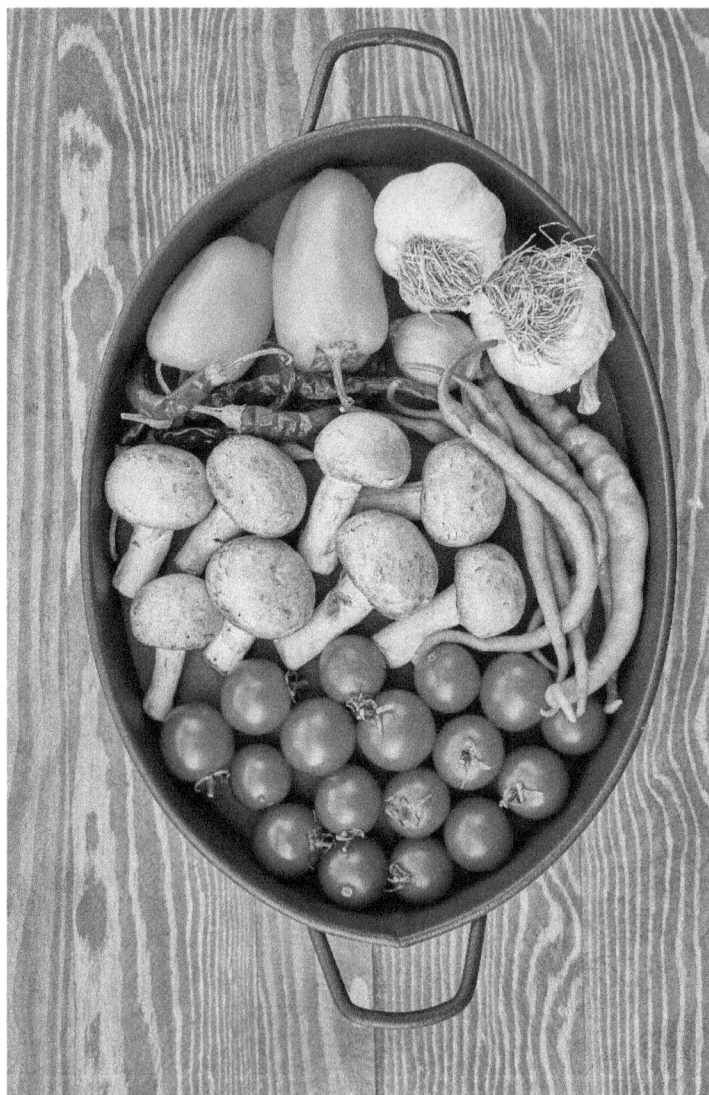

Marinated Trout

Ingredients:

small trout ready for cooking 1 glass of red wine 1/2 onion 1 clove of garlic 1 sprig of marjoram 1 tuft of parsley lemon juice flour salt and pepper a few lemon slices a few tufts of parsley

Description:

Chop the onions into half moons and garlic, parsley and put it on the bottom of a baking pan with high sides. Place the fish on top of the chopped mixture, and fill the pan with lemon juice (the trout must be completely immersed). Leave to rest for 24 hours with the help of a sieve. Filter the marinade and put the trout in a hot pan, add the marinade, filter and cook for 10 minutes over high heat.

Rabbit goulash

Ingredients:

1,200 kg rabbit 80 g ham 1 onion 1 tablespoon flour 1 clove garlic 1/4 l red wine 2 ladles broth 1 tablespoon paprika 2cl sour cream salt

Description:

Cut the conisglio into large pieces. Sauté the diced red onion and ham (if it is too dry, add 1 ladle of broth), flour the pieces of cone in the pan. Add all the spices you want, without exaggerating, salt and pepper to taste, add the sweet paprika and leave to cook for 30/40 minutes on a moderate heat with the lid on. At this point add the sour cream and leave to cook for another 5 minutes.

Tagliatelle With Ricotta Cheese

Ingredients:

- 350 g of tagliatelle
- 200 g of ricotta romana
- 1 tuft of parsley
- 1 pinch of marjoram
- 2 tablespoons of grated parmesan cheese
- 40 g of walnut kernels
- salt and pepper

Description:

chop the parsley and put it in a bowl with walnuts broken by hand, ricotta cheese, parmesan cheese, mix everything together until you obtain a homogeneous mixture. Bring a pot of water to a boil and add the pasta, when it is cooked, drain it, keeping a glass of cooking water, add the cooking water to the mixture and add the pasta to it.

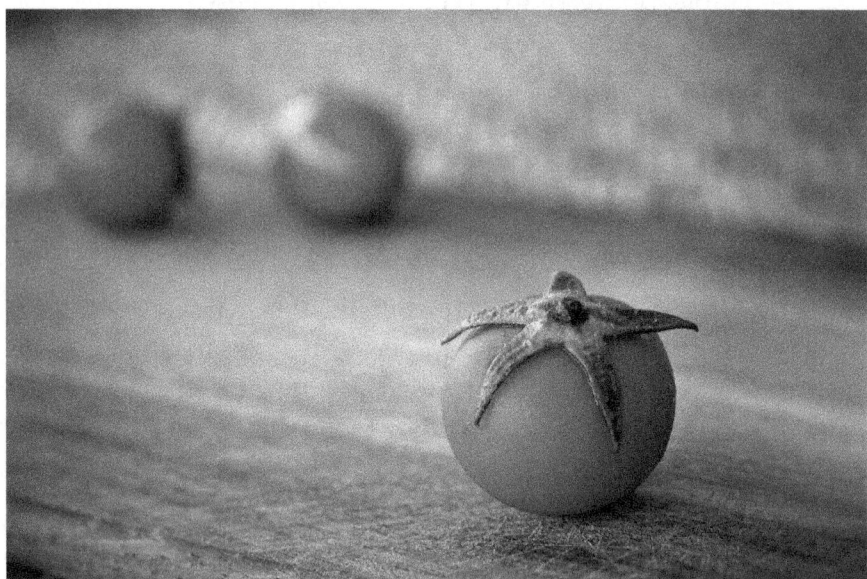

Mushrooms with baked potatoes

Ingredients:

4 potatoes; 400 g fresh mushrooms; 1 tuft of parsley; 1
clove of garlic
parsley; 1 clove of garlic; Parmesan cheese
grated Parmesan cheese; 2 glasses of milk; salt
of milk; salt; pepper.

Description:

Boil the potatoes in boiling water for about 45 minutes,
then drain them, let them cool, peel and slice them. In
the meantime, clean the mushrooms well with a small
knife and a wet cloth and slice them thinly.
Then finely chop the garlic clove and the parsley after
having washed them carefully and removed the stalks.
In an ovenproof dish, place a layer of sliced potatoes,
season with salt and freshly ground pepper and sprinkle
with a little of the chopped mixture and grated
Parmesan cheese. Then form a layer of mushrooms and
season it like the previous one.

Chicken with clay

Ingredients:

1 chicken 1/2 lemon 2 sheets of vegetable paper hard clay salt and pepper

Description:

Scorch the plucked chicken, clean them, wash and dry well. Lay it on a large sheet of vegetable or gamen paper. Inside the chicken put salt, pepper and lemon mesmo. Salt and pepper the outside of the chicken as well. Wrap the chicken in the paper, close it tightly at the sides and then wrap the package in the second sheet of paper. On the oven sheet or in a square cake pan place a layer of clay about three centimeters high, place the packet containing the chicken on it and cover this on each side with another layer of clay

three centimeters high. Place the preparation in a hot oven (about 200 °C) for 2 hours; when ready to serve, place the block of clay on a cutting board or metal plate and smash it with a hammer. Remove the paper, place the chicken on a plate and serve.

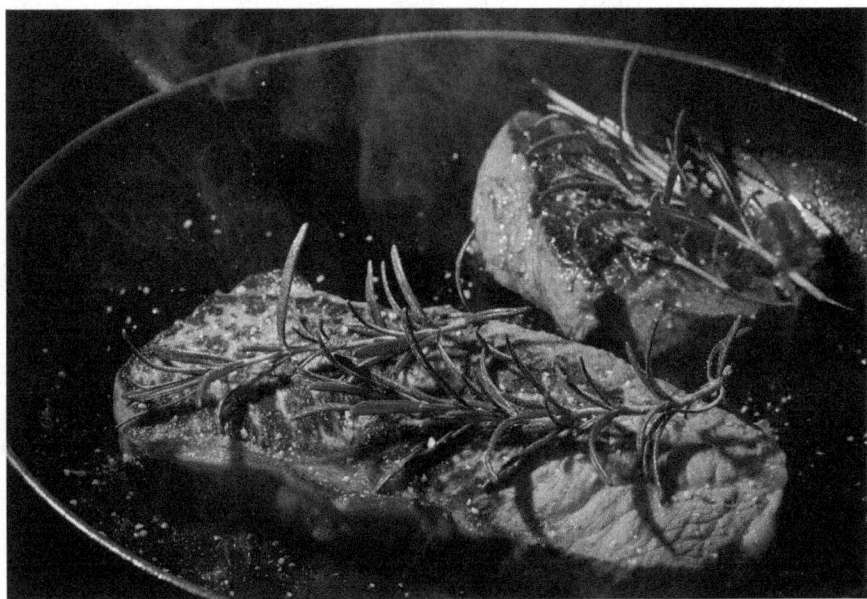

Mexican Veal In Jelly

Ingredients:

400 gr of sliced veal 80 gr of pork loin 80 gr of prosciutto half a clove of garlic (to taste) 50 gr of breadcrumbs - Milk one egg yolk grated lemon rind sage leaves one and 1/2 tablespoon of grated Parmesan cheese nutmeg - 80 gr of butter flour - a piece of cube for one liter of jelly salt and pepper

Description:

On the beaten meat slices, about 12x6 cm wide, spread with the blade of a knife the following filling: pass twice in the meat mincer the pork loin, the ham, the garlic and the breadcrumbs soaked in milk and squeezed; mix the egg yolk and the lemon rind, the Parmesan cheese, salt, pepper, nutmeg and mix everything well. Roll up the slices of meat thus prepared, put them together two by two with a sage leaf in between and stick them on two toothpicks.

Take care that the mexicans are well closed. Melt the butter in a pan, add the lightly floured Mexicans and let them brown on all sides. Pour in a little broth, cover and cook slowly for about 3/4 hour until the sauce has reduced. Remove them, place them on absorbent paper and let them cool completely. Arrange them in a deep dish and cover with the warm but liquid gelatin. Keep the dish in the refrigerator for a few hours before serving.

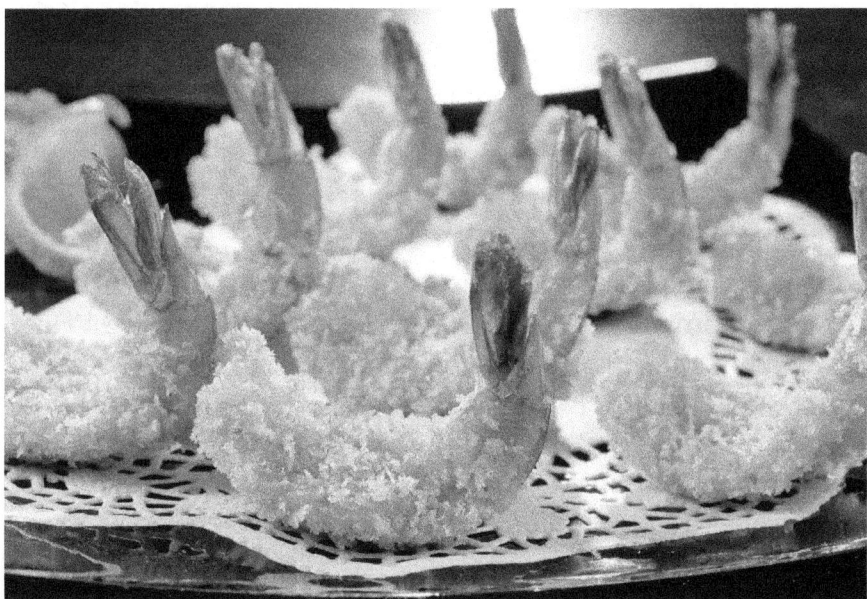

Summer chicken breasts

Ingredients:

- 4 chicken breasts
- 1 green bell pepper
- 1 tomato
- 2 salted anchovies
- 1 ladle of broth
- salt

Description:

toast the bell pepper on a grill and cut it into strips, cut the tomato into small pieces, season it and let it rest Heat a nonstick pan, when it is hot, put your chicken breasts, shake them and cook them well for a few moments, lower the heat and add the broth on the meat, let it cook for 10 minutes Serve hot accompanied by the tomato salad and grilled peppers

Veal With Creamed Yogurt

Ingredients:

- 800 g of veal rump in one piece
- 1 small glass of cognac
- sage; rosemary
- 1 ladle of stock
- 1 garlic clove
- 1 pot of yoghurt
- salt and pepper

Description:

put in a saucepan chopped rosemary, garlic and sage without frying, add the cognac and bring to a boil then add the meat and turn it on all sides cook for 1.5 hours adding the broth as soon as it is lacking after about 1 hour of cooking add the yogurt and leave the pot without a lid elapsed our hour and a half, cut the meat into slices and arrange on a platter serve with plenty of cooking sauce

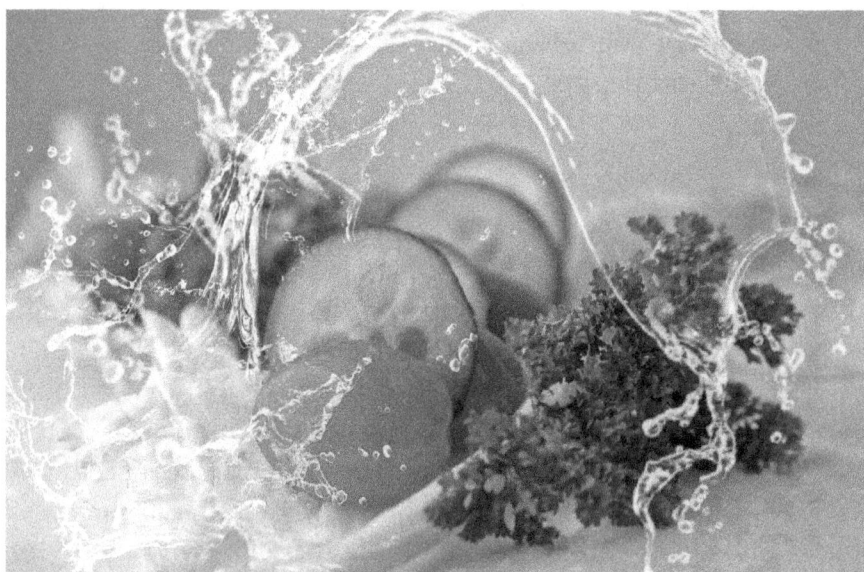

Roast With Walnuts

Ingredients:

- 600 gr of veal rump in a single slice
- sliced cooked ham
- 5 slices of cheese
- 60 gr of walnut kernels
- a tuft of chopped parsley
- butter or margarine
- 1/2 liter of milk
- salt and pepper

Description:

Beat the meat, lay the cooked ham, the cheese slices, the parsley and the chopped walnuts on top. Roll up the meat, tie it tightly so that the stuffing does not come out and brown it in a casserole with butter.

When the roast has browned on all sides, season with salt and pepper, sprinkle with milk and cook over medium heat for about an hour and a half so that the milk dries up

and the cooking liquid becomes creamy. Serve the roast cut into slices and covered with the sauce.

Summer Tomato Boats

Ingredients:

- 4 tomatoes
- 2 small cheeses
- basil
- salt
- white pepper

Description:

cut and empty the tomatoes and put aside the inside cut
the pulp of the tomatoes and add salt pepper and goat
cheese, add also some chopped basil leaves stuff the
tomato boats with the mixture serve with lettuce salad

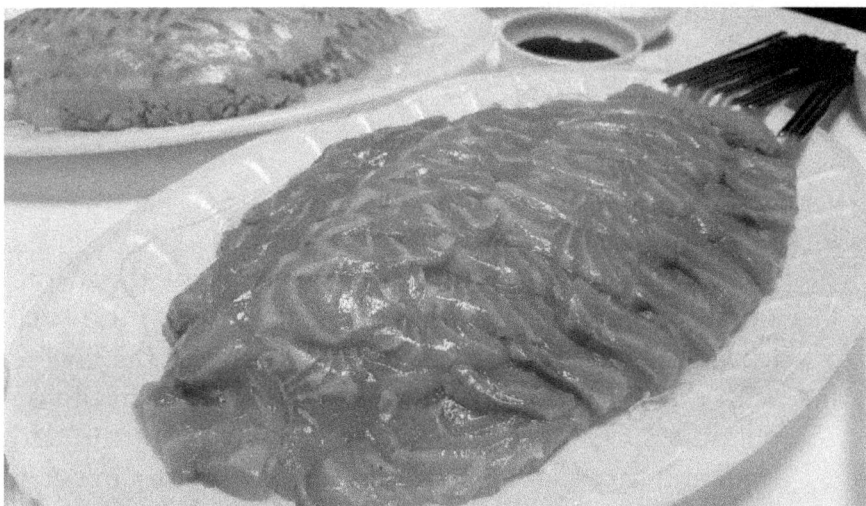

Appetizing Rolls

Ingredients:

- 8 fette of lean cooked ham
- 200 g of soft cheese
- green olives
- 1/2 ripe tomato
- basil ·
- 2 spoons of milk
- salt and pepper

Description:

Remove the stone from the olives and cut them into small pieces, dice the tomato and finely chop the basil leaves after washing them. In a bowl, mix the cheese with the milk and a pinch of salt and pepper until you obtain a spreadable cream, add the olives, tomato and basil and mix again. Spread the cheese mixture in equal parts over the slices of ham, spread it well and roll up the slices so that the filling remains inside. Serve the rolls on a serving plate garnished with salad leaves.

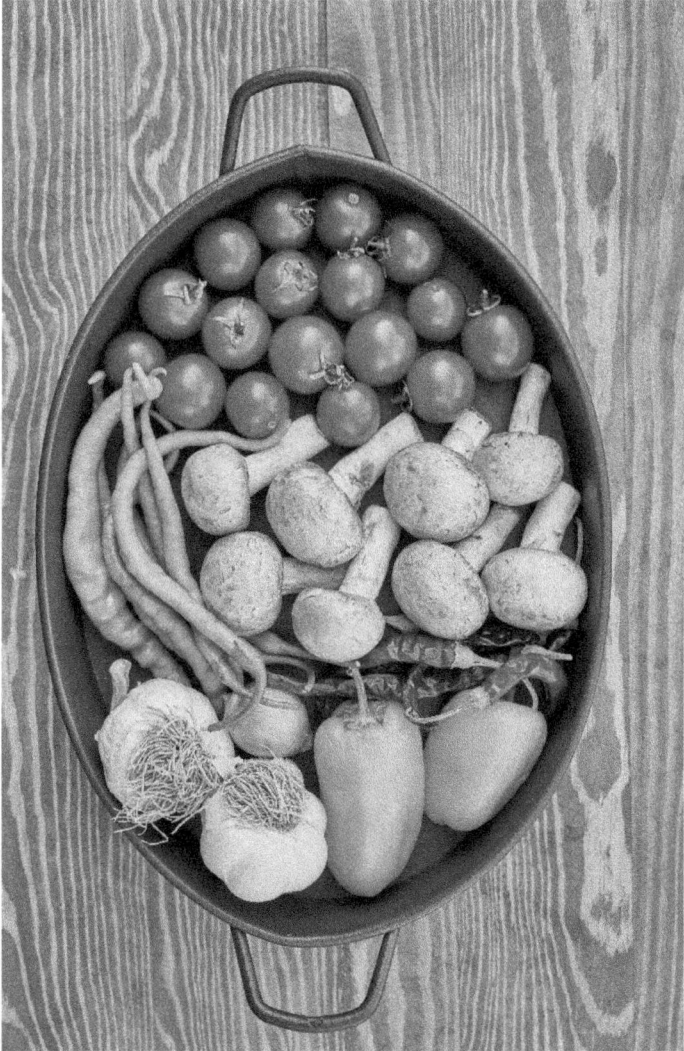

Tongue Salmistrata Croutons

Ingredients:

150 g of salted tongue 1/2 onion 300 g of boiled cauliflower tops 1 tablespoon of capers 1 tuft of parsley 1 small piece of stock cube 4 teaspoons of grated Parmesan cheese 4 slices of bread Salt pepper

Description:

Fry the chopped onion and add a glass of water and the stock cube. When the water has almost completely evaporated, add the tongue cut into slices and the cauliflower, cook for 15 minutes, then add a chopped mixture of capers, olives and parsley and continue cooking for another 5 minutes, turning from time to time.

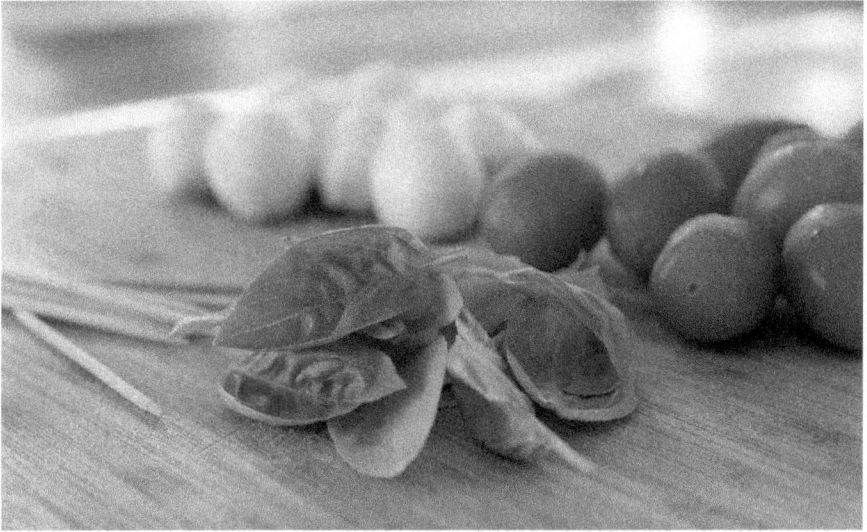

Mushroom Salad

Ingredients:

- 600 g fresh mushrooms
- 2 egg yolks
- parsley
- juice of 1/2 lemon
- 2 teaspoons of capers
- salt and pepper

Description:

Scrape the mushrooms with a small knife, removing the bottoms and soil, then wash them well with a damp cloth, without running them under running water because they would lose all their fragrance. Finally, dry them and slice them thinly. In a large bowl, place the egg yolks and, using a wooden spoon, beat them with the lemon juice, a little salt and a little pepper.

Carefully wash the parsley, remove the stalks and chop finely together with the capers. Add the chopped parsley to the eggs, pour the mushrooms into the bowl and stir well until the ingredients are well blended.

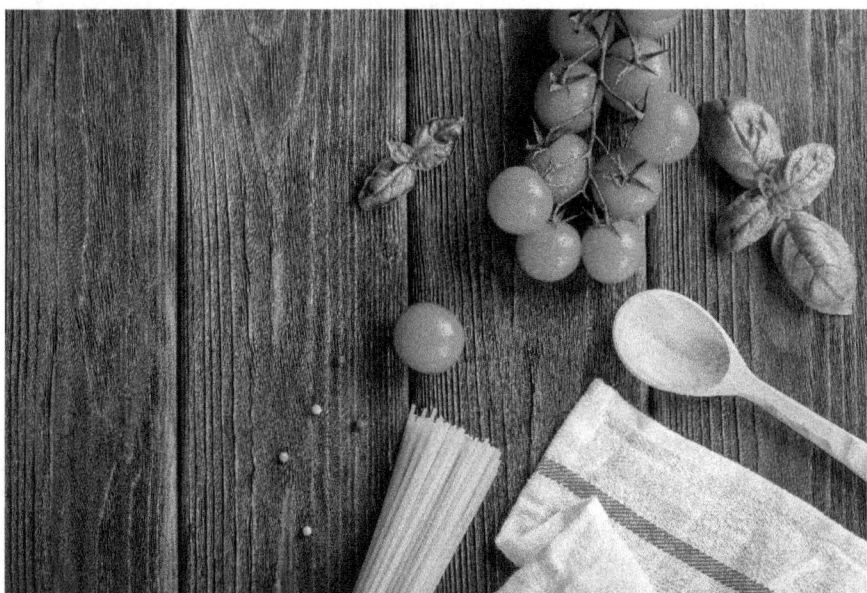

Ham Rolls For Kids

Ingredients:

- 5 slices of lean cooked ham
- 200 g of ricotta cheese
- 150 g of natural torno
- 1 handful of pitted olives
- 1 tuft of parsley
- 2 teaspoons of marsala
- salt
- pepper
- ready-made jelly

Description:

Chop the parsley and add the beaten olives. Separately, prepare the ricotta cheese with the tuna, add the parsley with the olives, salt and chilli pepper and mix until smooth and homogeneous. Lay the slices of ham and spread the mixture, roll the slices to form rolls and serve with fresh salad.

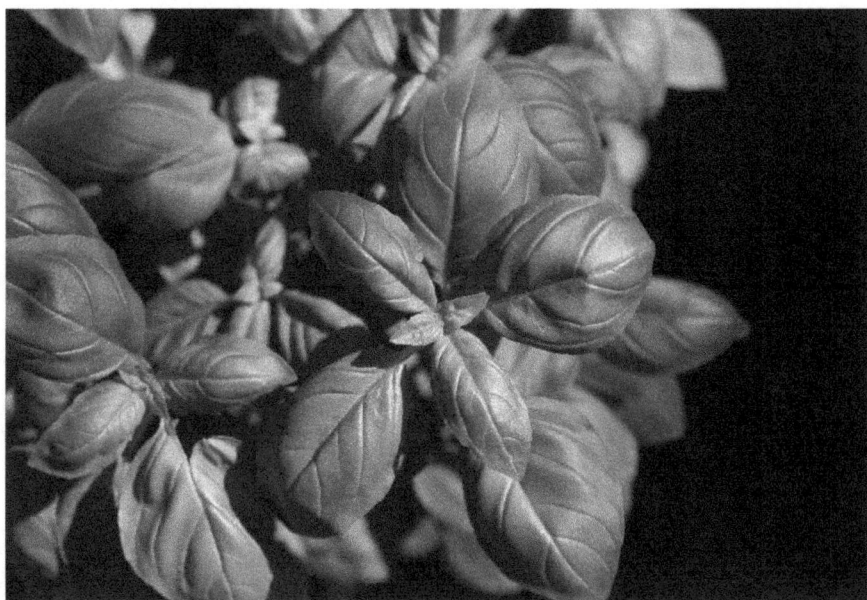

Fish Roulades

Ingredients:

4 fish fillets 1 garlic clove 1 sprig of parsley
2 anchovy fillets 4 tomatoes 8 teaspoons of boiled rice 1
bay leaf 1 ladle of stock, possibly fish stock 1/2 glass of
white wine salt pepper

Description:

chop the parsley, garlic and anchovies, dice the tomato and add
it to the mixture divide the mixture into 2 equal parts and
distribute them over the fillet roll up and secure with a
toothpick place the rolls in a saucepan, add crumbled bay
leaves wine and broth, cook for 25 minutes over low heat with
the lid on for the last 5 minutes, remove the lid and turn up the
heat

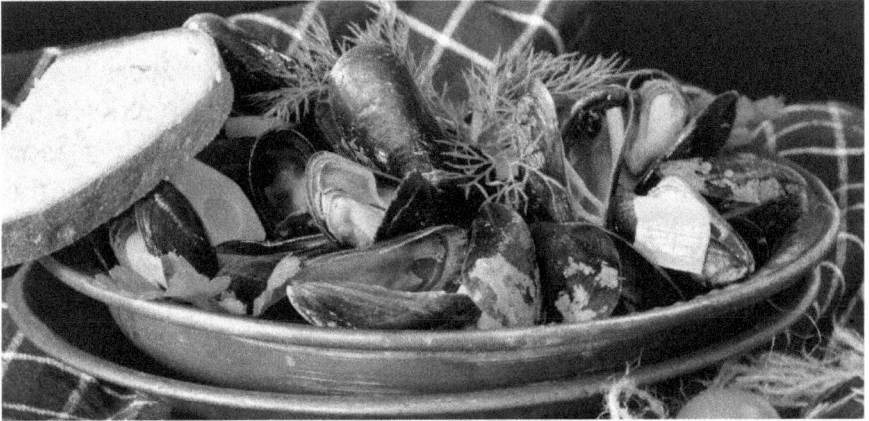

Pasta In The Oven With Artichokes

Ingredients:

350 g macaroni 4 artichokes I small onion 2 ladles of broth 1 sprig of parsley 1 mozzarella 30 g grated Parmesan cheese 6 tablespoons milk Salt pepper

Description:

clean the artichokes by removing the toughest leaves and slice them thinly Make a sauté of chopped onions then add the artichokes with a ladleful of broth, season with salt and pepper season the cooked pasta with the artichoke sauce in a baking dish place half of the pasta on hand create a layer of mozzarella frana hard-boiled eggs and ham and cover with the rest of the pasta, create a final layer of grated grana cheese and bake in the oven until a colored crust forms over the entire baking dish.

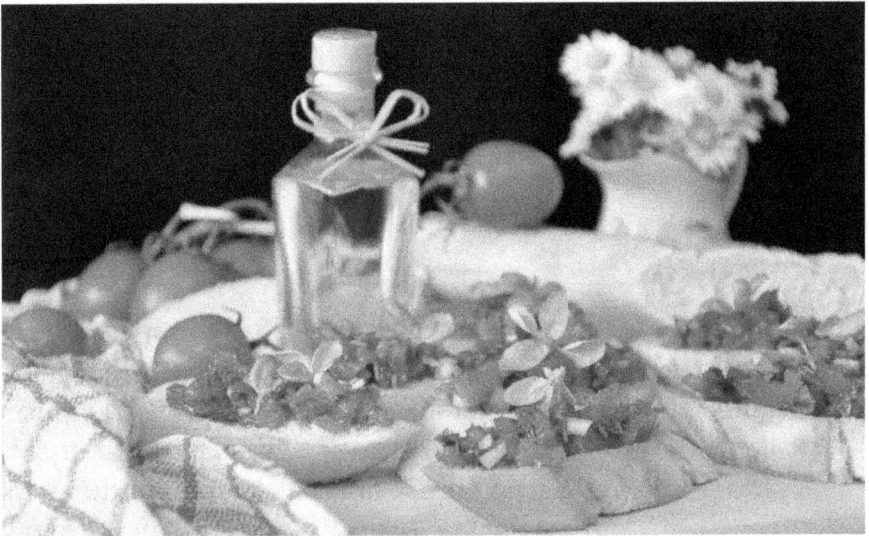

Leeks au gratin

Ingredients:

- 1,5 kg leeks
- 1 garlic clove
- 1 ladle of broth
- 200 g peeled tomatoes
- 1 chunk of parsley
- 20 g breadcrumbs
- 200 g grated Parmesan cheese
- salt
- pepper

Description:

Clean the leeks and cook them in boiling water for 20/25 minutes, drain them and place them in an oven dish, mince the garlic and parsley, dice the tomatoes and place them on top of the leeks, season with salt and pepper, add a layer of Grana cheese and bake for 30 minutes in the oven. (During the last 10 minutes of cooking, turn on the grill to create a golden crust.

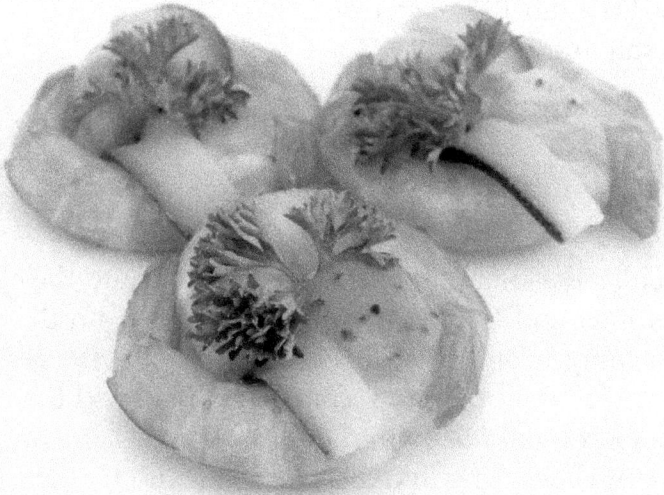

Asparagus Rice Soup

Ingredients:

- 200 g of rice
- 500 g of asparagus
- 1 sprig of parsley
- 1 spring onion
- 30 g of grated Parmesan cheese
- 1 egg
- 1litre and 1/2 of stock cube
- salt and pepper

Description:

Cut the asparagus into 4 cm pieces. Sauté the chopped onions and fry them with a ladleful of broth, add the asparagus and after a few minutes add the rest of the broth. When the broth comes to a boil, add the rice and cook it for about 15 minutes.
pour everything into the saucepan with the rice, turn up the heat and cook for 5 minutes, serve hot.

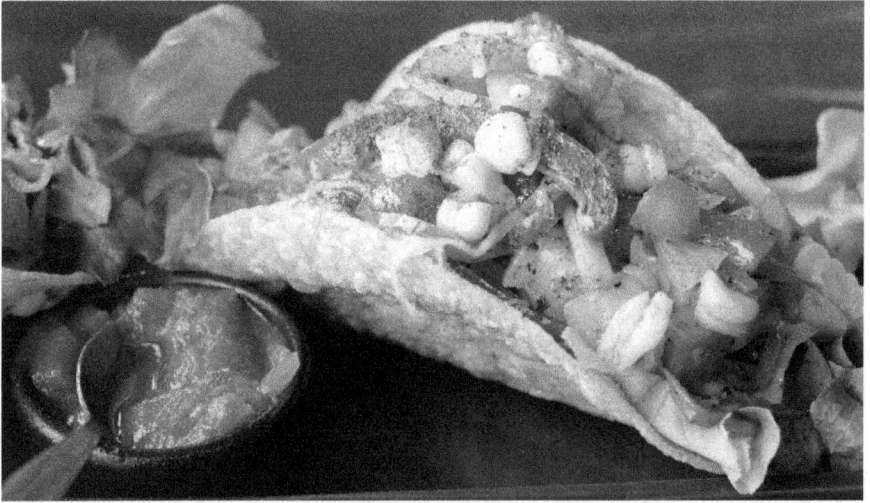

Spit-roasted fillet

Ingredients:

- 400g beef tenderloin
- Sliced bread
- 150g of bacon
- Sage
- Salt pepper
- butter

Description:

create squares of bread beef tenderloin and pork belly, alternate all elements on skewers. When all the skewers are ready, salt and pepper them and sprinkle them with melted butter, heat the oven or grill and cook for 30 minutes in the oven or 20 on the grill. Be careful not to let the sage leaves burn!
Enjoy your meal

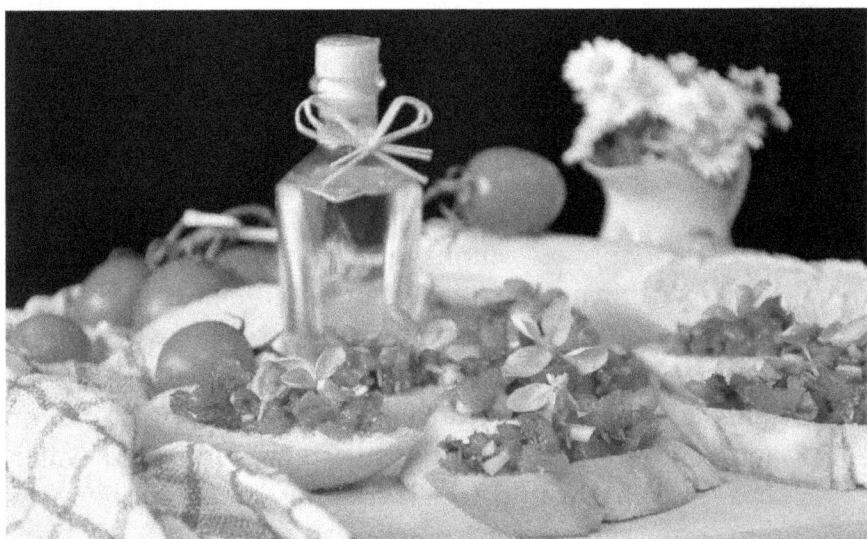

Kid Stew

Ingredients:

- 800g kid
- 500g Sardinian fennel
- 50g butter
- 50g bacon
- 1 onion garlic basil and parsley
- salt pepper

Description:

create a chopped onion garlic, parsley tomatoes and basil, put it in a bowl, separately cut into large pieces the kid, seasoned with butter and chopped bacon, fry until the meat becomes nice and golden, at which point add the chopped spices and tomatoes. Leave to gain flavor and remove from heat. Boil the fennel in salted water and drain halfway through cooking, add it to the meat and cook together for 1 hour, serve piping hot.

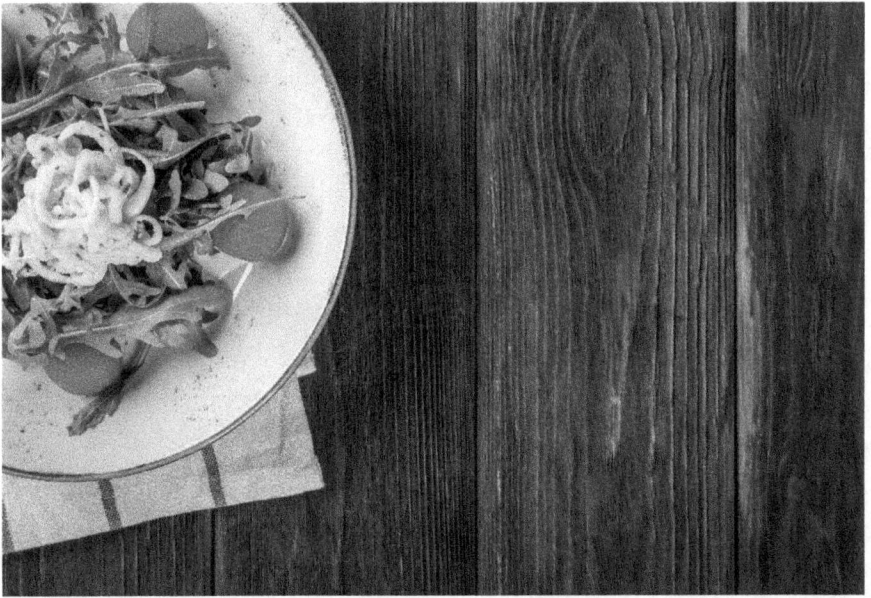

Stuffed Baked Potatoes

Ingredients:

800g potatoes 150g ground beef parmesan cheese provola garlic white wine oil salt pepper.

Description:

Wash the potatoes and cook them in the oven for 1 hour at 190 °, aside in a pan, saute the meat with a drizzle of oil and a clove of garlic; spent 1 hour, estaete the potatoes cut them in half and hollow them out to create small containers, with the stuffing of potatoes and meat and provolone cheese, create a mixture that we are going to insert in the potato shells, sprinkle with parmesan cheese and pass the potato boats in the oven 5 minutes with the grill.

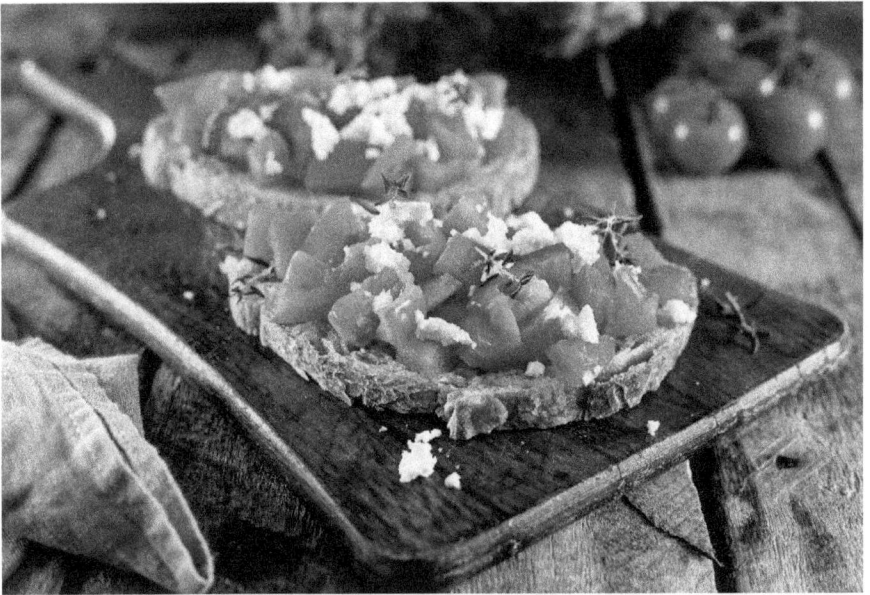

Orange Chicken

Ingredients:

500g chicken breast 50g flour00 2 orange butter 400g dates garlic thyme oil pepper and salt

Description:

cut the dates in half, salt and drain in a colander for half an hour; in a pan heat a little oil and a clove of garlic, add the tomatoes and thyme; separately squeeze the juice of 2 oranges; flour the chicken breasts and cook them in a pan, halfway through cooking add the orange juice, add salt and pepper, when the chicken is cooked, arrange it on a flat plate and accompany it with tomatoes .
Enjoy your meal.

Rosti

Ingredients:

750g potatoes 55g butter salt pepper

Description:

wash and put in a pot full of water the potatoes, bring to boil for 15 minutes, peel and slice into strips (help yourself with a grater multifaceted), salt and pepper, in a pan, melt a knob of butter, lay part of the potatoes and compacted making them adhere to the pan, after 2-3 minutes, turn it as if it were an omelette, the rosti should be crispy and colored
serve hot!

Rabbit And Pine Nuts

Ingredients:

whole rabbit 100g olives onions rosemary thyme garlic meat stock bay leaves pine nuts salt pepper

Description:

divide the rabbit into 5 pieces, brown it with a bay leaf and a sprig of thyme; sprinkle with a glass of red wine, then add the pitted olives, pine nuts and meat stock, cook with a lid on for at least 1 hour
serve in a nice serving dish with all the cooking juices.

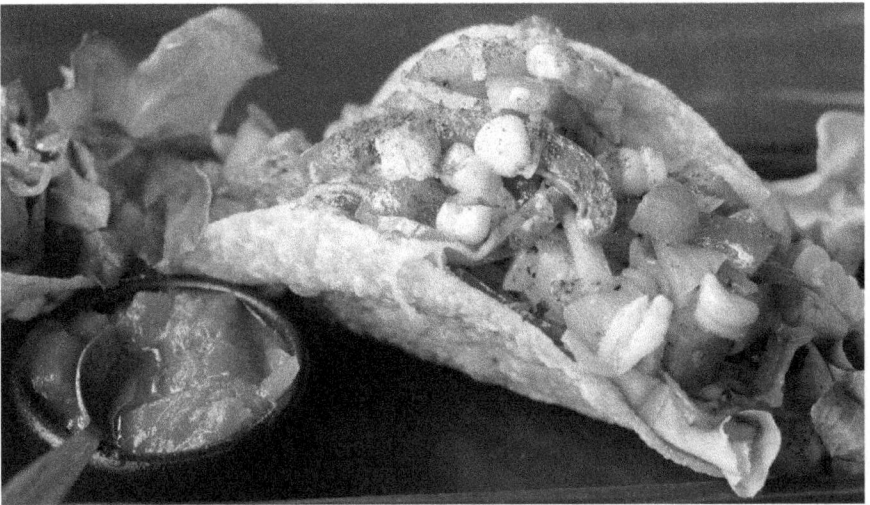

Beef Tagliata

Ingredients:

800g sirloin 100g arugula tomatoes salt pepper oil

Description:

Begin immediately to clean and cut the tomatoes, washed and cut the arugula and leave everything to one side, now take the sirloin and remove any filaments of fat, cook the sirloin for 3-4 minutes per side cu a plate rifata, compose the dish by putting the base of the arugula with tomatoes, above which adageremo the sirloin, cut into slices of ½ cm each.

Enjoy your meal!

Sea Bass And Olives

Ingredients:

1 sea bass onions carrots celery garlic 250g chillies bay leaves parsley salt oil pepper basil

Description:

create a diced with all the vegetables and place them in a pan with plenty of oil, aside clean the sea bass, scale and eviscerate it;
Salt the inside and insert a bay leaf and ½ slice of lemon, place it in the pan with the vegetables, 180° for 25 - 30 minutes, depending on the size of your sea bass.

Wet Prawns

Ingredients:

600g prawns 400g peeled tomatoes garlic chili pepper parsley salt and pepper

Description:

Carefully clean the prawns, remove the head legs and the black thread on the back, at this point heat a pan with a little oil and pan-fry for 1 minute the prawns, lower the heat and add the tomatoes, 1 teaspoon of granulated sugar and 1 cup of water, let cook with lid on for 5 minutes maximum, now uncovered raise the heat add the chopped parsley after 15 minutes, everything will be ready, serve with all the sauce that will be created in the pan
Enjoy your meal!

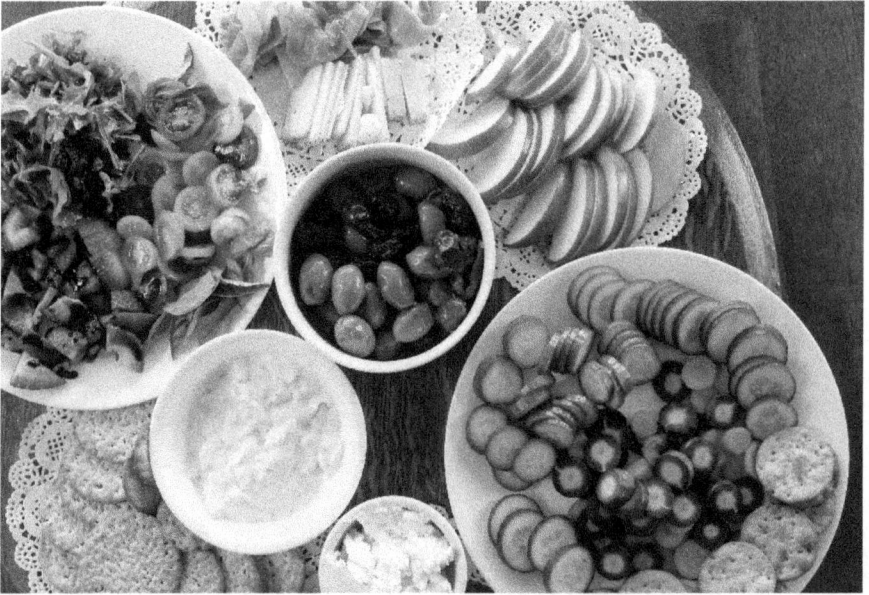

Mozzarella Fruit

Ingredients:

500g mozzarella 2 eggs milk flour00 breadcrumbs salt and pepper

Description:

Take the mozzarella and create equal cubes, leave them in a colander to lose all liquid, then pass the cubes in flour00, pass them in beaten eggs and finally in breadcrumbs, when the oil will reach 170 degrees, fry 3-4 pieces at a time, when they have reached a nice golden color, drain them from oil and place them on a piece of paper towels, serve immediately so at each bite will create the thread of mozzarella!
Enjoy your meal!

Vegetarian Cutlet

Ingredients:

450g zucchini 100g scamorza cheese breadcrumbs parmesan salt pepper oil 2 eggs

Description:

fry the zucchini and provolone, add the breadcrumbs and parmesan cheese, mix until you get a compact and smooth, from which you will get some balls that you will then make thin and give the shape of cutlet; at this point, in a dish, beat the eggs and dip one at a time your cutlets, pass them in breadcrumbs and cook them in a pan with a tablespoon of oil, when the cutlets will take a nice golden color, satano ready to be served
Enjoy your meal!

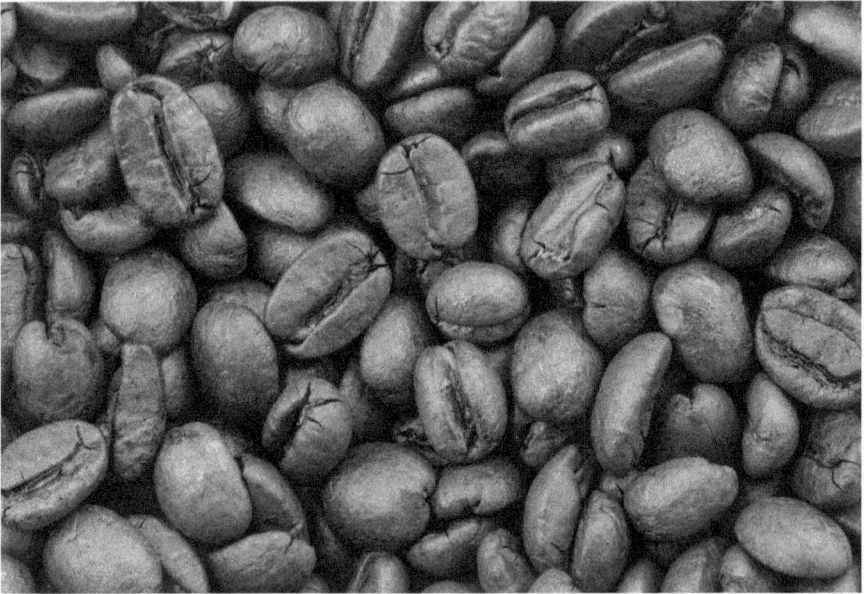

Rustic Eggs

Ingredients:

4 eggs 300g tomato puree 130g tomini cheese rosemary
oil salt pepper

Description:

cut cubes from tomini, aside in an oven dish, add part of
the tomato puree and line the entire dish, now insert the
4 whole eggs, add the cheese cubes and add the
remaining sauce; bake for 30 minutes at 180 °
serve piping hot with grilled bread croutons
Enjoy your meal!

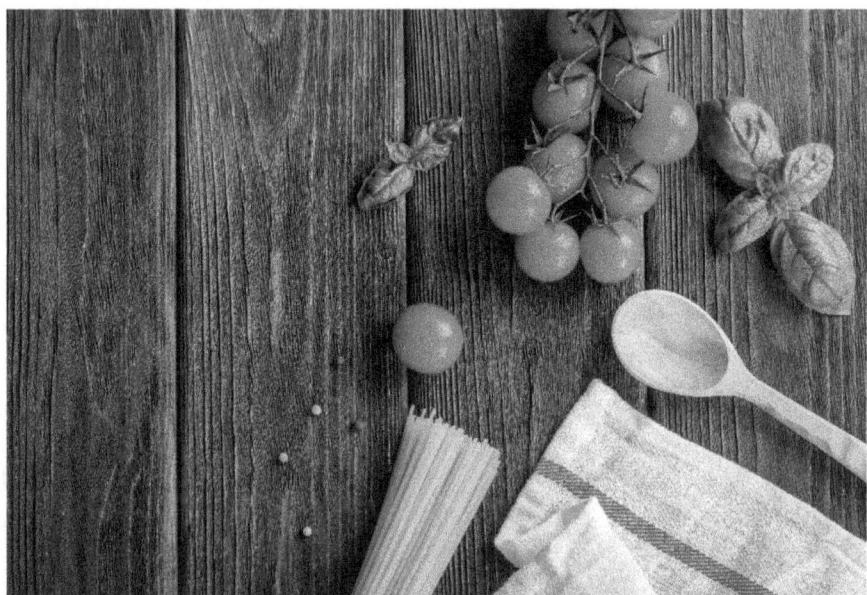

Pork Stew

Ingredients:

800g pork loin 450g potatoes celery carrots onion rosemary butter 800ml double malt beer salt pepper garlic flour

Description:

Cut the pork loin into cubes and flour them, separately grinded onion, carrots, celery and rosemary, in a saucepan melt a knob of butter and add the vegetables, let them stew and then add the pork and beer, close with lid, separately peeled and diced potatoes, after 40 minutes add them to the meat and cook without lid for 30 minutes on medium heat, when the cream is formed, plate!

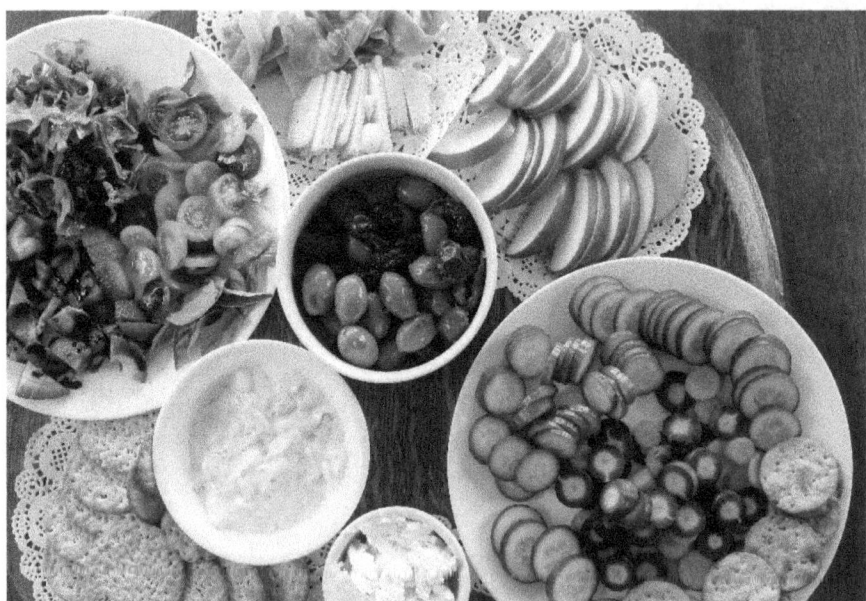

Sweet and sour pork

Ingredients:

400g pork carrots celery red and green peppers 150g pineapple onion oil flour00 baking powder pomooro sauce white vinegar brown sugar corn friend pineapple juice soy sauce

Description:

cut the pork into cubes, cut julien carrots peppers, create a batter with 80g of flour, seed oil and baking powder, dip each cube of pork and fry it, in a wok, fry the vegetables and pineapple into cubes 2-3 minutes will be enough, in a second wok, add the sugar laceto and soy sauce, add the pineapple juice, at this point add the vegetables and finally the fried pork, serve immediately, before the frying becomes soft
Enjoy

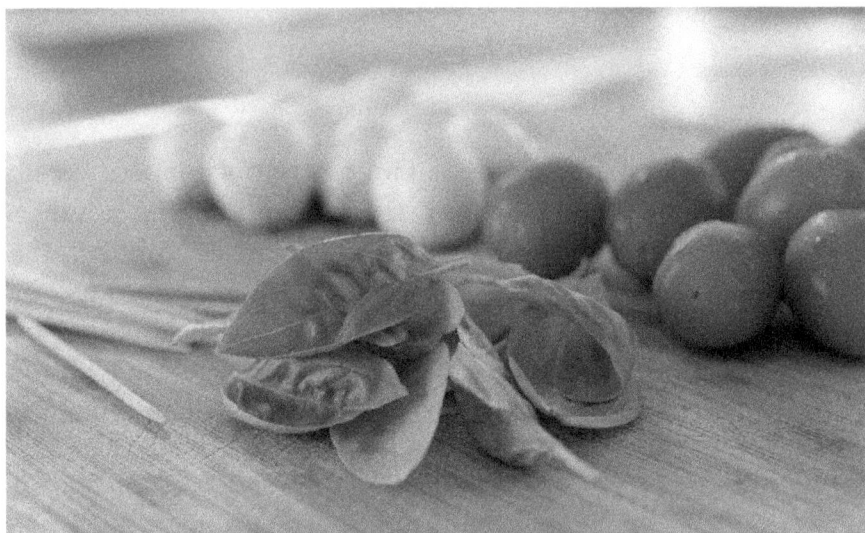

Gluttonous Chicken

Ingredients:

8 chicken thighs garlic paprika mustard rosemary thyme oil lemon zest orange zest polenta flour salt and pepper

Description:

Marinate in a bowl the thighs with oil, salt and pepper, add mustard, paprika, thyme and grated orange and lemon zest, mix and add the polenta flour, garlic, salt and pepper. Now take the chicken thighs and pass them in the spice mix and cook them in a pan with 2 tablespoons of olive oil.
Serve the crispy thighs immediately!

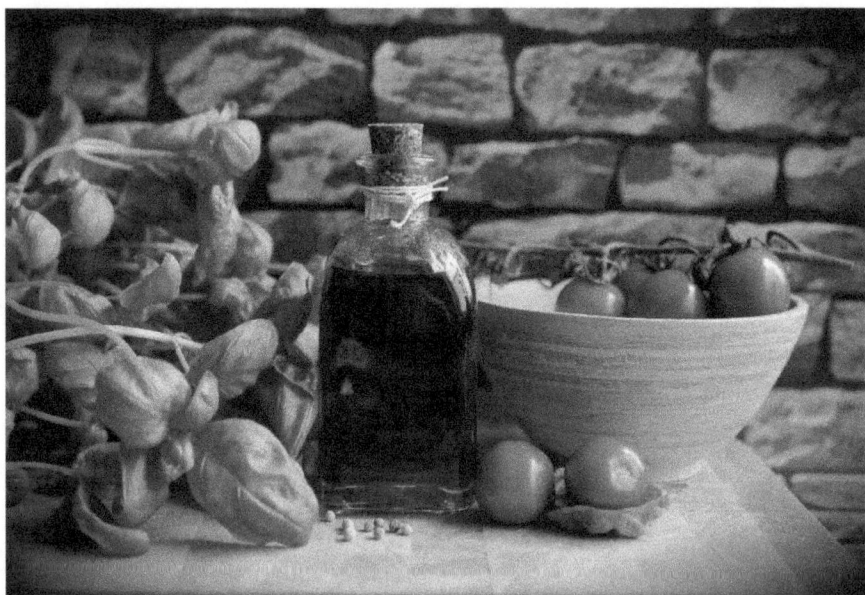

Irish Stew

Ingredients:

1kg beef (single piece) a can of guinness thyme black pepper salt 170g carrots paprika 2 tbsp flour00 oil tomato paste parsley garlic

Description:

Cut the beef into cubes put in a bowl with 2 tablespoons of oil; chop the onions and carrots, add flour and paprika and add them to the meat, brown 20 minutes the meat in an oiled pan and add quindiaglio onions tomato paste; insert in the pot also the guinness, cover and let it cook; after 15 minutes insert in the pot the carrots, cover for another 20 minutes, now the meat will be soft and tasty. Serve with mashed potatoes.

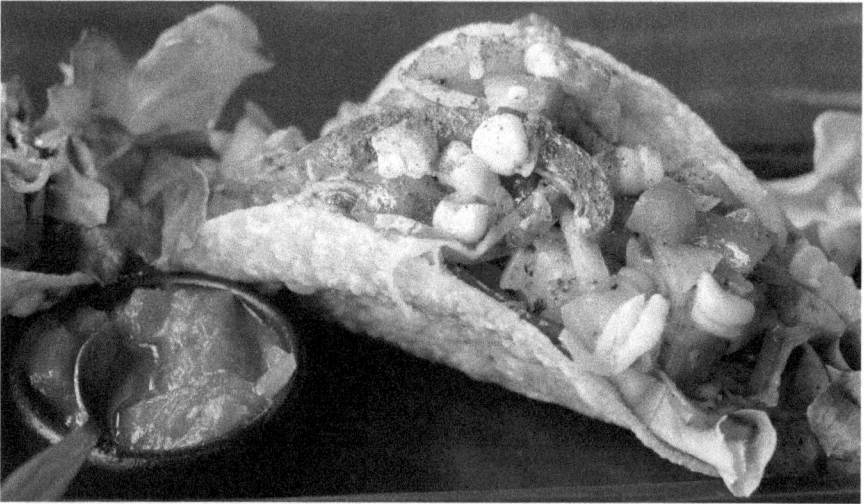

Stuffed Artichokes

Ingredients:

8 mammaries 1 egg salt pepper breadcrumbs vegetable broth parmesan garlic parsley 300g ground beef thyme

Description:

clean the artichokes and remove all the leaves until you get to the white ones, not to blacken the artichokes soak them in water and lemon, separately prepare the beef with 1 egg, breadcrumbs, Parmesan cheese and chopped thyme, add the garlic and breadcrumbs, mix everything, take the artichokes and open the heart in order to create a pebble that we are going to fill with beef, now we place the artichokes in an oven dish and bake for 30 minutes at 190 °.

serve immediately!

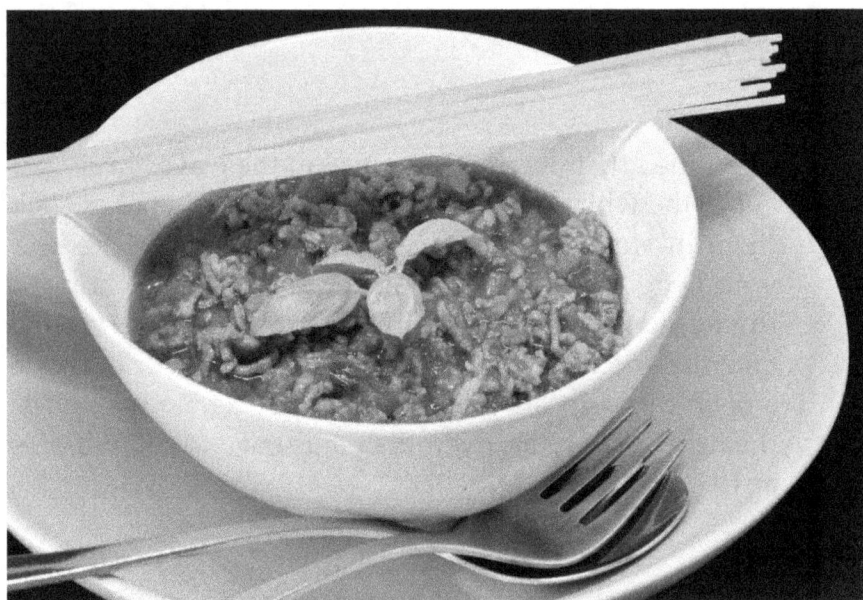

Crispy Chicken

Ingredients:

4 chicken breasts 100g corn flakes paprika 1 egg milk

Description:

in an oven dish put the cornflakes and crush them, add the paprika and mix; in a second bowl, beat the egg with milk and salt, then pass the chicken breasts first in the egg and then in the cornflakes; cook in a pan with 2 tablespoons of oil.
Serve with a nice seasonal salad or tzatziki sauce.

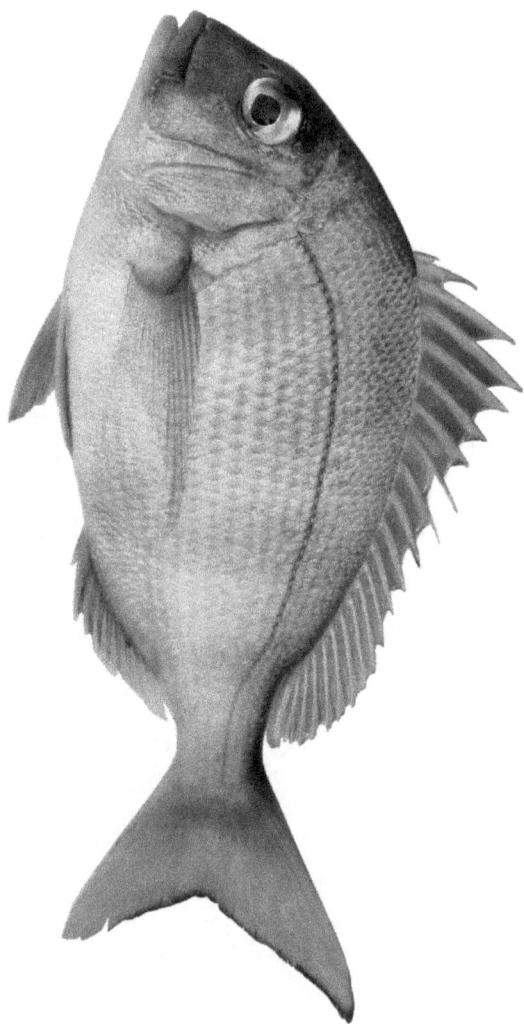

Baked Lamb

Ingredients:

800g lamb chops thyme rosemary peppercorns garlic oil zest of 1 lemon 500g potatoes

Description:

clean the chops so that the meat remains together and the bones are clean, let them marinate with rosemary thyme pepper oil and grated rind of a lemon, cover and let stand in the refrigerator from 3 hours up; peel the potatoes and cut them into cubes, season with salt and pepper and add the rosemary and oil; then take the lamb and transfer it to an oven dish with the potatoes; cover the rib bones with aluminum foil to prevent them from burning; bake for 1 hour at 200°.

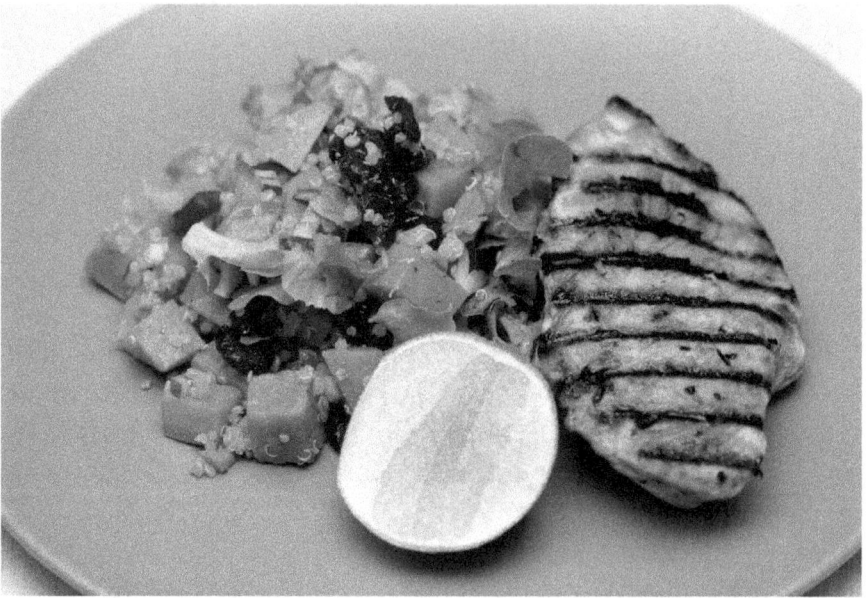

Rolled Chicken

Ingredients:

400g chicken breast pepper salt seed oil scamorza cheese slices spek rosemary

Description:

beat the chicken breasts in order to make them very thin, place on top 1 or 2 slices of provolone cheese, and also spek; roll everything and close the rolls with a toothpick, grill on the grill or on a ribbed steak pan until the chicken is well cooked

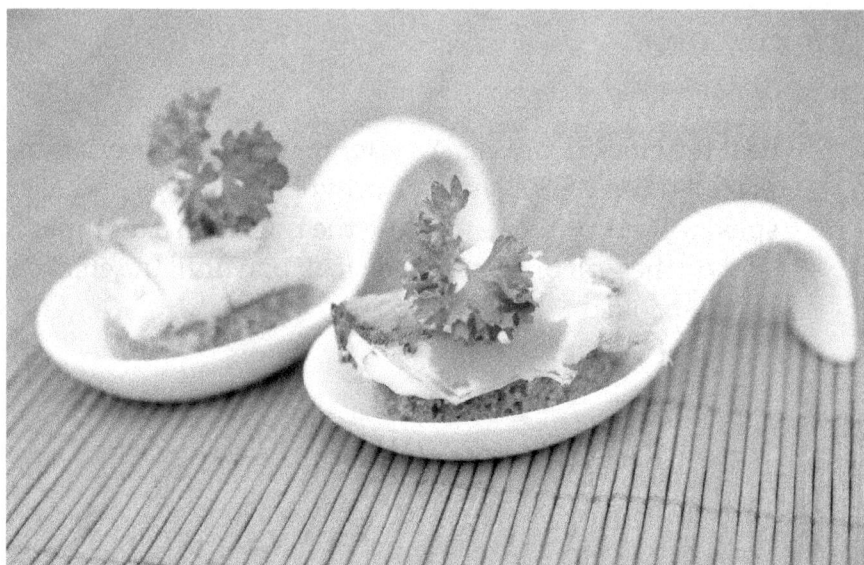

Pork In Wine

Ingredients:

400g pork tenderloin 300g red wine lemon zest shallot
50g butter oil pepper sage rosemary salt

Description:

Chop the shallot and dip it in red wine, rosemary, grated
lemon rind and butter; turn on the flame for 5-6 minutes;
tie the fillets and cook them in plenty of butter melted in
a pan, pepper and rosemary; when the fillets are ready,
plate them and drizzle with the filtered wine sauce.
Enjoy your meal

Veal Stew

Ingredients:

800g veal oil meat broth celery flour onions vinorosso salt pepper mushrooms mushrooms garlic parsley

Description:

in a pan wilt finely chopped onion, celery and carrot; after a few minutes add the veal already cut into stews; add flour and 2 glasses of red wine; cover and leave to cook over low heat; separately slice the mushrooms and pan-fry them with parsley; after 10-15 minutes, add the mushrooms to the veal, when the cream will have formed, the stew will be ready
Serve on a cold winter Sunday

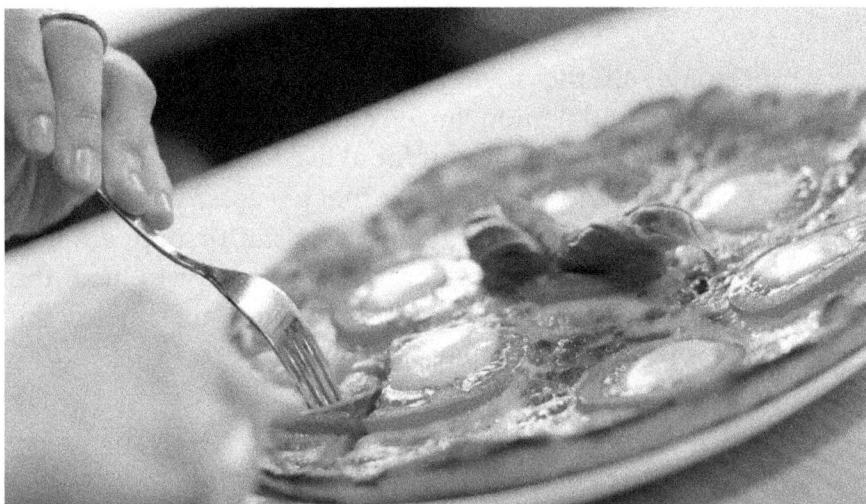

Grilled Meat

Ingredients:

pork chops pork chops sausage

Description:

marinate all the meat with garlic, oil, salt, pepper, rosemary and lemon juice, cover with cling film; let everything take on flavour for at least 24 hours; then turn on the grill and cook all the meat pieces, you can also add some vegetables such as zucchini or peppers and maybe create some skewers; be careful not to burn the meat pieces with too hot embers; you can accompany the meat with thathiki sauce
enjoy grilling!

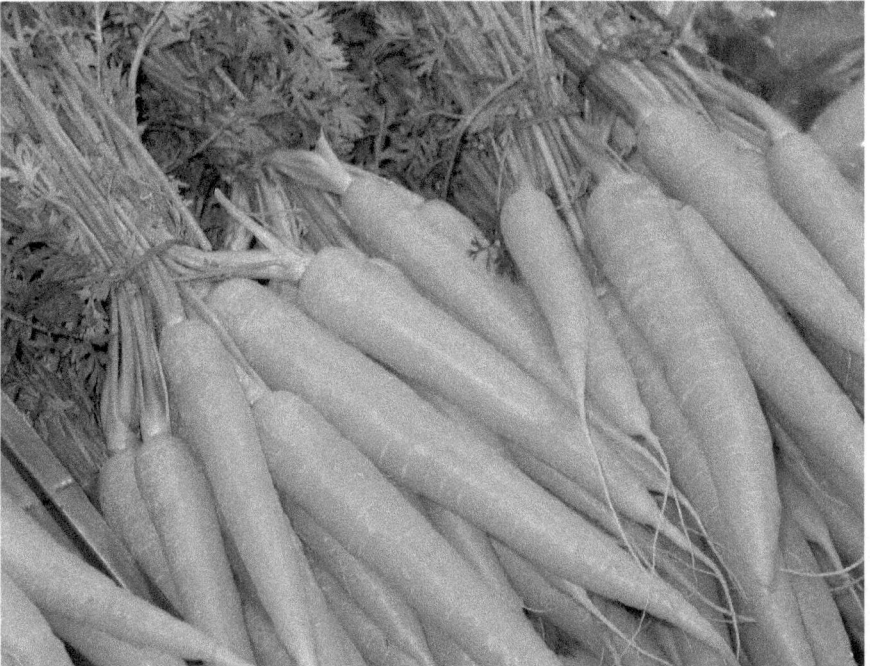

Cotechino And Lentichcie

Ingredients:

300g lentils 300g cotechino carrots celery oil bay leaves rosemary vegetable broth salt and pepper

Description:

soak the lentils for a couple of hours, separately bring to boil a pot of water and soak the cotechino for 30 minutes, then chop the celery, carrots and onion, fry them until no browning and then add the drained lentils, season with salt pepper and rosemary, open the cotechino and serve it in slices with lentils
Happy New Year!

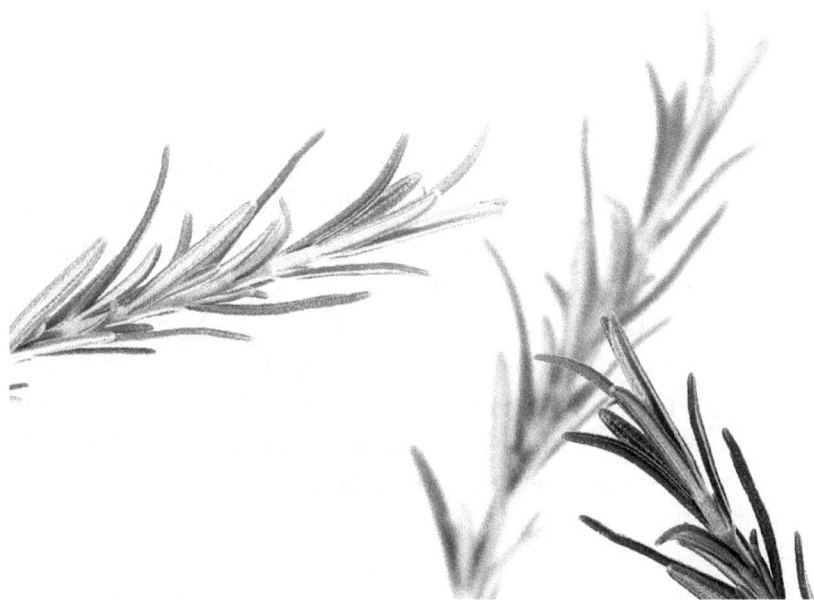

Milk Roast

Ingredients:

1kg of veal 1l of milk white wine butter carrots onions celery bay leaves pepper salt

Description:

bind the veal as a roast, separately in a mixer chopped celery onion garlic catore, in a pot capable enough melt 2 knobs of butter and brown the roast on all sides and remove it, in the same pot put the vegetables chopped before, when they are browned, insert the roast and milk, cover and leave on low heatoper a couple of hours; then remove the roast and cut it into slices; use an immersion blender to blend what remains in the pot; then serve the roast with its milk cream.

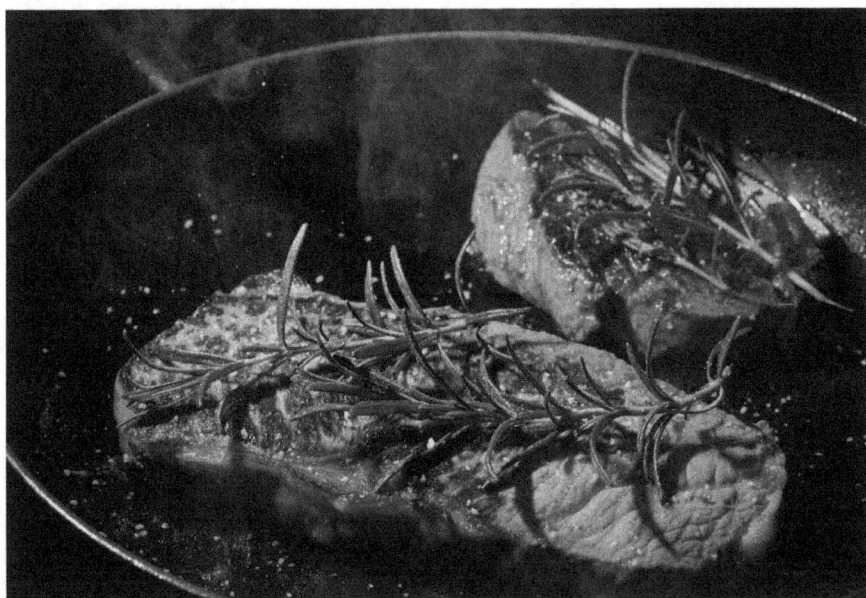

Country Rabbit

Ingredients:

1kg rabbit onions oil sage rosemary chili pepper garlic
400g tomato puree salt pepper 500ml broth

Description:

Clean the rabbit, in a pan with a tablespoon of oil brown
the chopped onion with chilli, rosemary and sage, now
add the rabbit cut into 5-6 pieces, add the broth and
puree, cover and cook over medium heat for 20 minutes,
turn occasionally, if you like you can also insert the
entrails of the rabbit in the pan, toast the croutons of
bread and serve with rabbit.

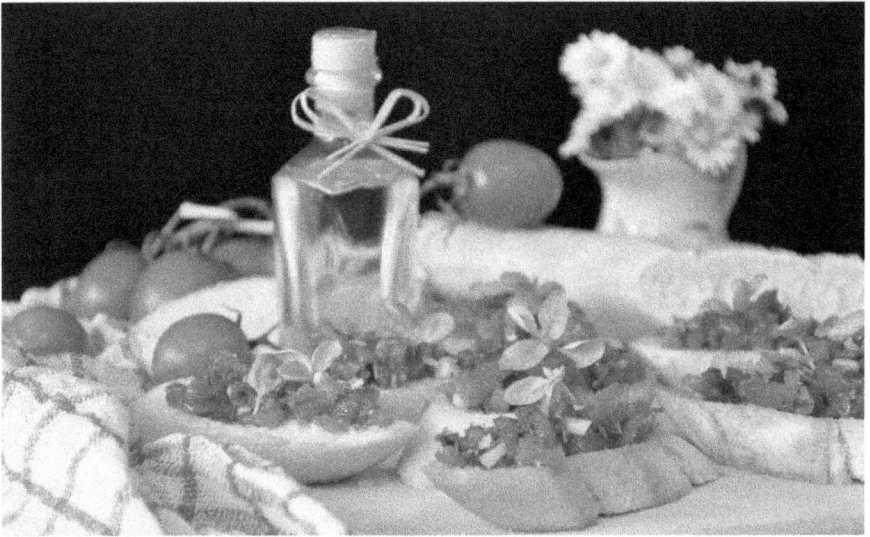

Cod Fillets

Ingredients:

600g cod 50g pine nuts butter 50g farin00 salt pepper parsley

Description:

Toast the pine nuts in a nonstick pan and keep them aside, in the same pan melt 80g of butter, separately combine the flour with pepper, then flour the fillets and cook them in the pan with butter, aciugateli from excess oil and keep them aside, in the same pan add 150ml of water chopped parsley pine nuts and wait until the water has evaporated, serve your fillets with the sauce just pulled.

Sardines A Beccafico

Ingredients:

500g of sardine's bay leaves breadcrumbs raisins parsley
piinoli anchovies sugar salt pepper oil honey

Description:

in a bowl put the raisins with cold water for 10 minutes,
aside in a pan pour 1 tablespoon of oil and toast the
breadcrumbs, chopped parsley anchovies and add them
to raisins drained with pine nuts and salt; then arrange
the sardines, spread the mixture on each of them and roll
them up, blocking them with a toothpick, place them in
a greased oven dish, 25 minutes in the oven at 200°.

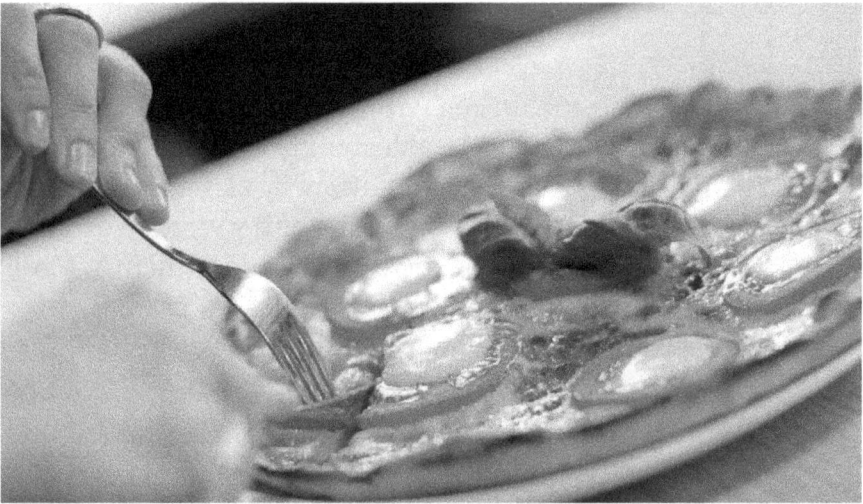

Tripe Parmigiana

Ingredients:

1.5kg clean tripe onions oil meat stock parmesan salt pepper 200g tomato puree

Description:

Chop the onion and brown it in a pan; cut the tripe into strips and put it in the pan for 6 minutes; add the tomato puree, broth and parmesan cheese and cook for 20-30 minutes; a variation could be to add cannellini beans to make our recipe even more rustic.

CPSIA information can be obtained
at www.ICGtesting.com
Printed in the USA
BVHW092207310521
608489BV00013B/1862

9 781802 760538